YOU
Can Live
In
Divine
Health

YOU
Can Live
In
Divine
Health

Joyce Boisseau

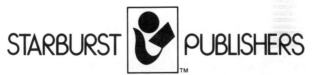

STARBURST PUBLISHERS

P. O. BOX 4123, LANCASTER, PA 17604   (717) 569–5558

Other Books By Starburst Publishers:
Devotion In Motion by Joan Hake Robie
A Bucket Of Finger Lickin's by Joan Hake Robie
To My Jewish Friends With Love by Christine Hyle

For information about *Devotion In Motion Seminars* and
other products by Starburst Publishers write:

Starburst Publishers
P.O. Box 4123
Lancaster, PA 17604

ISBN: 0-914984-02-0
Library of Congress Catalog Card Number 82-60240
Printed in the United States of America

In dedication to:

Our Lord Jesus Christ,
Whose blessed guidance and inspiration
impressed my spirit with these words herein;

and to

My husband Larry, whose love and
encouragement enabled me to record
what my spirit heard.

CONTENTS

PREFACE

One of the most controversial issues facing the evangelical community today is that which is developing over sickness and divine health. The position is taken by some that all one has to do to have divine health or spiritual healing is make the proper "confession." They believe that it does not take prayer and fasting, obedience, waiting on God, or a holy life. You need only "confess it" and "you've got it." While "confessing the Word" and being "positive" is all well and good, there is much more to it. There are many churches throughout the county, packed to capacity, that have weekly healing services, but the sad truth is that the majority of faithful believers go home without a sign that their prayers have been heard.

What misery, doubt, sense of unworthiness, and confusion must plague those who do not receive the healing for which they prayed. It is the knowledge of the plight of these people, over the past fifteen years, which led me to months of prayer, hours of searching the Scriptures, fasting, attending countless healing services, medical seminars, and psychiatric workshops and visiting hospitals. My search led me many miles from home and into almost every denominational church, from charismatic Catholic to interdenominational prayer groups conducted in private homes. There is one theme which seemed to emerge time and again, whether in a general hospital, rehabilitation center, psychiatric hospital, mental health group therapy session, or prayer for healing in church services — *we make ourselves sick and are reluctant to be made whole.*

In order to be whole and healthy the problem must be approached at its point of origin — the spirit man. Medicine alone cannot cure an affliction which is caused by the turmoil, resentment, and disharmony of the inner self. The cause of the physical condition has to be discovered within the emotional nature of man and dealt with in a problem-solving manner which will bring about a transformation within. *This is the only way any of us can be permanently healed, whether by faith or by science.*

This relationship between the soul and physical illness is termed "psychosomatic illness," indicating an imbalance affecting both the soul and the body. The illnesses suffered by most of mankind illustrate that *we cannot expect to have good health without a right relationship with God.* If we are to enjoy physical and mental health we will need to understand the laws of the universe which govern us and the consequences of living in violation of them.

My research also revealed that our illnesses and afflictions are *multi-dimensional.* If we are to be wholly well, we will have to come to an understanding of all that is involved in our sicknesses and begin working to right ourselves at the root cause.

Research into causes of psychogenic disorders reveals that illness and disease are most often meted to us by our consciences. This active element of judgement, which is an essential part of the soul, determines, for us, what is right and wrong. There is evidence to indicate that *the soul then chooses the kind of punishment from which the mortal self will best learn to act in accordance with the laws of God.*

Dr. Helen Flanders Dunbar (MIND AND BODY: PSYCHO-SOMATIC MEDICINE copyright 1966, Random House) says: "The chooser of the symptoms does not set out to get sick with malice aforethought. There must be a real emotional need for illness first. Then on the borderline between the known and the forgotten, the choice of symptom will be made.

Before it does permanent damage to the body, the emotional need for illness must be removed. It can be done only if the victim first understands what has roused the need and faces up to the situation. Self-understanding is not the most pleasant experience in the world, but it may be worth the price. It may help to remove both cause and symptom."

Although the subject I have chosen for this book may be somewhat controversial, I believe it is a timely one. Watching the trends developing over the past fifteen years, I have found that the people of our country have slid into twelfth place by the world's standard of health. Currently, the debate over the Christian's inherited right to divine health is about ready to erupt and become a divisive factor in the Body of Christ. It need not be so if Christians will search the Word for deeper truth beyond that offered by teachers who stand for or against "faith confession." Moving between the two realms, I offer medical and spiritual considerations concerning the dilemma of sickness, and hope to lead the reader to a new understanding that, in the area of his own health, there is much more for which he can and should assume personal responsibility.

I

Is There Any Sick Among You?

We are living in the most exciting era of mankind since Adam and Eve were driven out of the Garden of Eden! Our life expectancy limit has been extended to the point that senior citizens now make up an ever increasing percentage of our population. Our infant mortality rate has been decreased. Immunization serums have eliminated the threat of many childhood diseases.

Intricate surgery gives a second chance to those with cardiac problems; deteriorated hip joints can be replaced with plastic; vital organs can be transplanted from a donor; radiology can eradicate all traces of cancer in some people; and psychotropic drugs keep mentally ill people functioning in society. Research continues in major laboratories around the world where discoveries of new combinations of chemicals make possible, in the near future, the prevention of major organ deterioration.

But visions of health and long life do not stop with the field of medical science. To the contrary – we see evidences everywhere that certain of mankind have caught sight of the vision of perfection which God intended when He placed man in Paradise. Health!

Not by single units, but rather in groups of hundreds, people are breaking chains of bondage which have held civilization captive with the *idea of sickness.* FAITH in the Word of God is dawning in the human heart like spring sunshine after a long, dark winter — faith to believe in health and healing and in life more abundant!

This newly awakened faith peers over a horizon of negativity, fear and unbelief; its golden rays of Spirit-inspired wisdom cutting asunder the dark shadows of our long night.

"Besides this you know what hour it is, how it is full time now for you to wake from sleep. For salvation is nearer to us now than when we first believed; the night is far gone, the day is at hand." (Rom. 13:11-12, R.S.V.)

Through faith in Christ, people from every walk of life are stepping forth to claim healing of their afflictions. Healing services are a regular weekly function at many churches. Ministers and elders are fulfilling the direction given in James 5:14: *"Is any sick among you? let him call for the elders of the church; and let them pray over him, anointing him with oil in the name of the Lord: And the prayer of faith shall save the sick, and the Lord shall raise him up; and if he have committed sins, they shall be forgiven him. Confess your faults one to another, and pray one for another, that ye may be healed. The effectual fervent prayer of a righteous man availeth much."*

The faithful believers in my home church became representative of fifteen years of study of similar people, the world over, who sought spiritual answers to human ills: physical affliction, addictions, financial limitations, marital discord, emotional imbalances, family difficulties and unemployment.

The testimonies I heard from those who had experienced positive results from prayer triggered in my memory the many inspiring stories I had heard in similar meetings since this research began. The enthusiasm and zeal were inspiring:

- A fifty-year old woman was healed of breast cancer;
- A man in his seventies dramatically waved a white cane which he claimed he no longer needed because his sight had been restored;
- A young woman told of a malignant brain tumor which had disappeared after a year of fervent prayer!
- Another woman, a laboratory technician, who was diagnosed as having Hodgkins disease, is back at her job — whole, vibrant and healthy after three years of waiting on the Lord in complete faith of her deliverance!
- A young mother was released from the hospital so that her wish to die at home with her family could be granted. She had cancer of the spine and the prognosis given was to live only three more days. She was instantaneously healed during a Sunday morning service.
- A man in his late fifties was given the last rites of his church. His cancer-filled lungs were beyond operation or chemotherapy. A prayer group interceded on his behalf that fateful night and he was healed!
- A young man was converted to Christ after surviving

27,000 volts of electricity! He is now the pastor of a church.

— A fibroid tumor disappeared without a trace in one woman who was awaiting surgery; a middle-aged man had a kidney condition healed and stones disappeared! Several thyroid imbalances were corrected; three people under psychiatric treatment were made whole and no longer needed psychotropic drugs.

— A young mother told of her year-old baby being born blind because of a milky film over his eyes. She took him to a healing service and as the minister laid hands on the child, the film slid off his eyes onto his little cheeks.

Certainly, such testimonies serve to increase the faith of believer and doubter alike. The pastor of one congregation claimed that at least half of those who came forward for healing received that for which they had prayed.

Then why is it that others would come forward, week after week, asking for prayer for the same condition, with no positive result? Many from this group became confused and bewildered by the seeming inconsistency in the ways of God and they would fall from the faith, disappointed and embittered.

Many of the people who regularly attend healing services today are being influenced by the current "positive faith confession" teaching which is gaining ascendancy in evangelical, charismatic circles. The belief is that all one needs to do to have divine health or spiritual healing is make the proper confession of faith. Then, there are the evangelists for whom healing is not a matter of divine judgment. They say it is God's will for all of us to be completely healthy at all times. Because Jesus overcame sickness and sin at Calvary there is no reason for any of us to be sick. The charisma of some of these late-rising expounders can sway an audience of thousands but are their claims scriptural? Furthermore, are the followers actually being healed and living in the divine health which they claim? If not, then, why not?

Scripture says, *"If ye have faith and doubt not . . . "* (Matt. 21:21), *"And all things, whatsoever ye shall ask in prayer, believing, ye shall receive."* (Matt. 21:22) Again, Scripture promises, *"If thou canst believe, all things are possible to him that believeth."* (Mark 9:23) Or . . . *"What things soever ye desire, when ye pray, believe that ye receive them, and ye shall have them."* (Mark 11:24) Certainly, these Scriptures taken alone would indicate that healing is a promise we have the right to claim. Why, then, do they not work for everyone? Why are some healed and others overlooked?

It is too easy to say that the person who didn't receive healing lacked faith. How much faith does it take to be healed? *"As a grain of mustard seed,"* (Matt. 13:31) we are told. Someone counters, "Ah, but his faith must have waivered." I am immediately reminded of the father of the epileptic child who said, "I believe! Help thou mine unbelief!" Someone else then enjoins, "His faith obviously wasn't founded upon Jesus Christ!" In my mind's eye I see Peter approaching the Gate Beautiful where the man who had been born crippled sat begging alms. When Peter saw him he didn't ask if he believed in Jesus Christ or if he had faith. He simply said, *"Look on us"* (Acts 3:4) — and in the name of Jesus of Nazareth the man was instantly and completely healed! But the favorite explanation of the positive-faith confession group is, "God already had answered prayer and healed that man. He just didn't receive!"

According to some recent studies, *born-again* Christians have better health than the average churchgoer, and when they do succumb to illness or are involved in accidents the healing is faster and the recuperation period shorter. These are generally optimistically inclined people who view illness as a part of life, however unpleasant, which must be approached as any other situation which challenges them. They are matter-of-fact about it, seeing it neither as God's judgment against them nor as a martyrizing experience.

And there is another faction within the camp of born-again believers, however, who take a far different view. Sickness is sin, a violation of the trust placed in their hands when Jesus suffered and died on the cross. They have no more right, according to their teachers, to participate in sickness than they do in overt lawlessness. When sickness does befall them they are overcome with shame and condemnation, unable to expose or confess it. They may even refuse any kind of medical help, insisting that would be a show of the smallness of their faith. They use the Scriptures as their unfailing promise that if they just believe hard enough and hold on tight enough, the healing will eventually come. My mind recalls how, when I was twelve years old, a nine year old playmate was injured while playing. The mother, refusing medical help for the child, stood on prayer for the boy's healing. He bled to death before morning!

Spiritual healing is a fact. There are too many miraculous cases on file, the world over, certifying the reality of divine intervention, for anyone to casually state there is no such move of the Spirit of God today. I can testify to that fact. Over the years my family has had six healings of major importance. Once, in the last split second of a crisis, I was brought back from the very mouth of death. But, you ask, "What about those who are not healed? What about those who died believing, until the end, that their healing would come?"

The media loves to pick up on "religious cult" exploits, mocking the endeavors of the sincere while hindering the growth of the Body of Christ. For that reason, we need to be thorough in our study of Scripture and wise in our application of it. We must be careful that our teaching is not a stumbling block and does not put another into bondage. In this hour, the Bride of Christ is being commanded to prepare herself for her Bridegroom and to present herself without spot or wrinkle. The divisiveness, which is sprouting because of a difference of opinion concerning healing and divine health, must be stopped. Teachings on the Holy Spirit should edify *all* believers, not just a certain few who are projecting a horizontal "health, happiness, prosperity" regimen while ignoring the vertical bar of the cross which portends suffering, sacrifice and tribulations.

In the months during which I was doing research for this

writing, I was led to many healing services conducted by some of the most famous evangelists gifted in the healing ministry. I studied the teachings of nearly every nationally known Bible teacher, attended medical and psychiatric seminars, did volunteer work in hospitals, nursing homes, rehabilitation centers and a mental health transitional program. My search was for the answer to the haunting question, "Why do some people continue to suffer with their affliction, despite prayer and faith, while others are healed?" I traveled many miles from home, into almost every religious denomination, from charismatic Catholic to interdenominational prayer groups conducted in private homes. One theme which began to emerge was:

There are Scriptural promises which give birth to belief in absolutes . . . the complete and perfected Plan of God "on earth as it is in Heaven." However, mankind has not yet come into that perfection. In this incomplete and separated state, we are constantly being influenced at levels of consciousness of which we are not even aware. Furthermore, we have inherited traditional beliefs of sickness and suffering from the collective unconscious of humanity just by being part of the human race. These thought patterns and unconscious attitudes aren't easily disposed even by those who are aware of them.

We must take note that the Word of God speaks to all people of every age – past, present and future, and is meant to edify all believers. All things considered, we might have to concede that with our present limited vision we cannot know the mind of God. Even the most intense investigation by the most avid researcher will leave vital questions unanswered so that we are left to say with Paul, *His grace is sufficient unto me.* (2 Cor. 12:19 Paraphrased)

That is not to say that sickness is an accident or that health is a coincidence. There is an ordered and divine purpose to the seeming chaotic confusion of our mortal lives. At times, though, the sensibility of these human experiences and the continuity of the working of God seems all but lost. Were we able to view the pattern taking shape in the tapestry of our personal history, we would observe a definite design unlike that of any other. It is inherently our own and by faith we must believe that *"all things work together for good to them that love God."* (Rom. 8:28)

Another truth which began to emerge as I poured over Scripture, thumbed through dusty medical journals, digested articles in psychiatric periodicals, listened to the personal confessions of countless men and women, and absorbed case histories from psychological profiles was: *"For our light affliction, which is but for a moment, worketh for us a far more exceeding and eternal weight of glory. . . ."* (2 Cor. 4:17)

Scripture proves that we are in the process of being perfected. It appears that our life's experiences have been ordered by us because of the deficiencies of our mortal nature and unfinished ego. Most of us have called into existence the trials which beset us because our personal circumstances are the most expeditious means by which God can teach us to trust in Him. We have brought upon ourselves the consequences of our rebellious actions as well as rewards for obedience, and that each of us eventually learns through the pleasure/pain syndrome and that we are bound by what we have created; that is, until we realize the lesson being taught. We then come to the understanding . . . at every level of our consciousness . . . that God is The Sovereign Ruler of this universe and we must be obedient to His commands.

To lament that we are not free-will agents and have no control over our experiences is to confess that we believe God is pernicious and inconstant by nature, meting favors or punishments to whomever He randomly chooses. On the other hand, do those who expect to receive blessings because they have spoken a positive faith decree or produced a certain formula from Scriptures (possibly lifted out of context) reduce Almighty God to a *genii in a magic lamp,* a practice which borders on magical incantations? Consider a branch of "Christian" teaching which developed this theory in the early 1900's. It is known as "mind science Christianity" and is extremely dangerous to the unsuspecting ones who are lured into it because of being promised "the good life." In time and practice, Jesus Christ loses the central position in the church and man is exalted to that position. This kind of philosophy can be the forerunner of Humanism. Christian teachers who veer off in this direction are wandering onto dangerously thin ice because of that initial temptation to use the power available to call into manifestation all that which he desires. *"For the time will come when they will not endure sound doctrine; but after their own lusts shall they heap to themselves teachers, having itching ears; And they shall turn away their ears from the truth, and shall be turned unto fables.* " (2 Tim. 4:3)

Did Paul, James and Peter indicate by their exhortations that those who accepted the gospel were *always* going to be divinely healthy and never encounter problems once they were baptized into the Body of Christ? And, did they speak of a hundredfold return on whatever was given to the furtherance of the ministry? Note that they did caution, *"Thou therefore, endure hardness, as a good soldier of Jesus Christ."* (2 Tim. 2:3) *"But watch thou in all things, endure afflictions."* (2 Tim. 4:5) *"despise not thou the chastening of the Lord, nor faint when thou art rebuked of him: . . . "* (Heb. 12:5) *"Take, my brethren, the prophets, who have spoken in the name of the Lord, for an example of suffering affliction, and of patience."* (James 5:10) *"Beloved, think it not strange concerning the fiery trial which is to try you, as though some strange thing happend unto you. . . . "* (1 Pet. 4:12) *"Wherefore let them that suffer according to the will of God commit the keeping of their souls to him in well doing, as unto a faithful Creator . . . "* (1 Pet. 4:19) *"Humble yourselves therefore under the mighty hand of God, that He may exalt you in due time . . . "* (1 Pet. 5:6)

Is it realistic to expect, even demand, that life be a bed of roses? And, let us consider the trend of some, not all, faith confessing believers, who think that they can behave as spoiled children, before an Almighty God, with the petulant order, "Father, you promised it, and I demand now . . . in the name of Jesus . . . that you honor that promise!" I have seen grown men and women stomp their feet and actually shake their fists at heaven as they put forth these forceful petitions! What happened to, *"For ye ought to say, If the Lord will, we shall live, and do this or that."* (James 4:15) or *"Humble your-selves in the sight of the Lord, and he shall lift you up."* (James 4:10)

Realistically, sickness is on the earth. It affects the right-eous, the holy, the innocent, the young, the old, the mother, the father, the president, the pope, the kings and princes, the rich and the poor, the high and the lowly, the beast, the fowl and the fish, the soil, the air and the water. The earth is cursed with sickness! It has been since Genesis 3 when God cursed the ground because of Adam and Eve's disobedience. And all of us who are of the earth are subjected to that curse, regardless of our spirituality, and must wait — even as Paul said in Romans 8:21-23, *"For the creature itself also shall be delivered from the bondage of corruption into the glorious liberty of the children of God. For we know that the whole creation groaneth and travaileth in pain together until now. And not only they but ourselves also, which have the first fruits of the Spirit, even we ourselves groan within ourselves, waiting for the adoption, to wit, the redemption of our body."*

The curse will be ended when the new heaven and new earth are come: when the first heaven and the first earth are passed away. *"And God shall wipe away all tears from their eyes; and there shall be no more death, neither sorrow, nor crying, neither shall there be any more pain: for the former things are passed away."* (Rev. 21:4) In the meantime we suffer from childhood diseases, seasonal colds, the ravages of aging, the stings of insects, the bites of poisonous vipers, sunburn, frost bite, hay fever, poison ivy, brackish water, epidemics caused by viruses and germs, not to mention the ecological pollution caused by man himself.

Scripture reveals to us the other sources of sickness and affliction as the breaking of health laws (Leviticus): the judgment of God (Psa. 199:75; Neh. 9:33; Ex. 15; Dan. 9:14; Mic. 7:9; Luke 23:40 and Acts 13); taking communion unworthily (1 Cor. 11) and from Satanic attack or oppression. But, basically, all of these original sources of sickness began and are perpetrated by man himself in the form of personal sin (James 5:14; Rom. 5:12; James 1:14; Psa. 38:3; Rom. 7:5 and many more).

As we observe the explicit order of the universe which bears silent testimony to the precision of God's creation, we realize the very atoms of our bodies are microscopic replicas of our solar system. Each of us is a tiny atom in the structure of the whole and when we begin to vibrate out of harmony temporarily, adjustment must be made within us to stabilize and correct our awkward motion to bring us back into harmony with the rest of creation. This process is taking place constantly throughout the cosmos in every kingdom of creation: animal, vegetable, mineral; in the planetary system and in the internal life of man himself. Sometimes the adjustment which must be made with mankind to bring him back into harmony appears as an affliction. We may bemoan our "misfortune," but time proves that we had been looking through a glass dimly and very frequently the Lord has proved the truth of the saying that,

when we grieve in the flesh we are at the same time rejoicing
in the spirit, for another fetter very well may have become
broken at that time! David said, *"It is good for me that I
have been afflicted; that I might learn thy statutes."* (Psa.
119:71)

Even though we don't see this process taking place and acknowledge it as an internal force which is working to perfect
us, it is consistent throughout our lives, for believer and
non-believer alike. It is impossible for any one of us to upset
the balance of our Perfect God's creation. It is absurd and
impossible!

A case in point is the issue of "gay rights" which has
brought so much notoriety in our country lately. One news-
paper article stated that a new disease has been discovered
among homosexuals which has no known cure and it has
killed 70 percent of those diagnosed with it. Herpes II is a
new veneral disease without a cure. Apparently, people can
write new manuals on moral ethics, but if the soul can
not live with it, the body is certainly going to suffer the
consequences!

So who do we upset when we are out of balance with the
perfect order of the Kingdom of God? The answer is, ourselves, and those individuals close to us who permit our
perfidious behavior to also disrupt their peace.

The mores of society may change, people can develop
"liberated" moral viewpoints, but the Great I AM THAT
I AM never changes. The guidelines God established at the
dawn of creation are in force yet today, for believer and
unbeliever alike. We cannot ignore Him out of existence

and thereby escape His judgment of our actions.

Atheists and agnostics receive just recompense as *"the reward of unrighteousness"* (2 Pet. 2:13a) as do those intellectuals who view our Father as little more than a concept of superior power of archetypal human need.

And what about those who profess Him and stoutly defend their belief while continuing in their committment to carnal activities? Too often their actions shout so loudly no one can hear their testimony!

We become aware that God Almighty must be more than the god of our religious inclination. He must be God of every action and thought we entertain if He is to be able to effect changes and healings in our lives and bodies. Until He becomes Lord Omnipotent of all that we are, we are the children of the father of this world, heir to this kingdom of sin, sickness and death.

Then, how does all this effect those who are born again of the Spirit of God, who believe with faith that they are redeemed from the curse and that *"by whose stripes ye were healed?"* (1 Pet. 2:24) Is there no hope for health and happiness on this earth — not even for the believers?

When we rightly divide the Word of God, reading such "faith Scriptures" in the context inspired by the Holy Spirit, the message is clear and uncompromising: *"Forasmuch then as Christ hath suffered for us in the flesh, arm yourselves likewise with the same mind: for he that hath suffered in the flesh hath ceased from sin; That he no longer should live the rest of his time in the flesh to the lusts of men, but to the will of God."* (1 Pet. 4:1) *" . . . that we, being dead to sins, should live unto righteousness; by whose stripes ye were healed."* (1 Pet. 2:24b)

Scripture affirms that our afflictions are to correct, to chasten, to instruct, to teach righteousness, to purge, to turn us toward God, to perfect faith in us and to bring us to glory. For most of us the procedure would be less arduous and not so repetitive if we would only remove the spiritual blinders and see the cause of our afflictions, instead of looking so diligently for something or someone to blame!

So many of us go through life like the oxen at the primitive grist mill, just plodding along with our heads down, endlessly turning the wheel, following mindlessly upon the heels of the ox in front of us, never awakening to the fact that, although we are moving, it is only in a small circle and we are repeating the same exercise over and over again. We hurt, but we don't know why. We suffer, but we blame and accuse rather than question. An example is a woman who complained to her doctor recently, "My stomach hurts terribly when I push on it like this!" The doctor stoically retorted, "Then quit pushing on it!"

If we refuse to realize that we cause much of our own pain, we defer that moment of spiritual awakening and its subsequent growth. And, naturally, we delay that stage of our development when good health is the norm rather than the exception.

Until we become awakened, we are "bound by the law," the law of cause and effect. *"Therefore all things whatsoever ye would that men should do to you, do ye even so to them: for this is the law and the prophets."* (Matt. 7:12 also see

Luke 6:31; Gal. 5:14)

Our experiences appear to be happenstance. We act and react and are acted upon while we continue as blind recipients of whatever "fate" bestows. It needn't be this way. The exciting manifestation in this latter day rain is seeing the Word of God springing into life and power in the life of the believer so that he is awakened to the promises of God and the authority *He has given us power to use the name of Jesus Christ to take control of our circumstances.* We weren't meant to be useless flotsam and jetsom on the sea of life, being buffeted about with every wave and wind. We are promised, " *I will instruct thee and teach thee in the way which thou shalt go: I will guide thee with mine eye.* " (Psa. 32:8)

The awakening of the wisdom of God cannot come to us unless we are born of the Spirit of God. Until that time, we continue in oblivious blindness or we seek out intellectual, scientific or occult answers. This wisdom of God is foolishness to us until we are born of His Spirit and can perceive spiritual things. For many, wisdom is gained as the result of intense physical or emotional suffering. To others, it is the reward for diligent religious disciplines. Still others claim to have been "awakened" in a moment of abstract concentration when they became cognizant of the self's inherent unity with all other creation. Without the inner witness of the Holy Spirit most of these people develop a heretical doctrine!

Peter refers to the spiritual awakening, *"as unto a light that shineth in a dark place . . . the daystar arising in your hearts: . . . "* (2 Pet. 1:19b) The "light" is the Word of God illuminating the inner self — the soul — with the truth which sets men free.

When we receive that truth, we are no longer bound by the curse of the law, if, and when we begin to take responsibility for the effects of the law of sowing and reaping. The "truth" also sets us free from the desire to sin or transgress, because inwardly we comprehend that we cannot act in violation to the Law of God. What is meted shall be measured again and again.

As we begin to realize this fundamental truth of all life we begin to measure our thoughts, feelings and actions against the measuring stick of perfection — Jesus Christ — and we make the decision regarding what our lives shall be. **If we don't want sickness we can have better health by following the directives given in the Word of God.** We learn that when the "inside of the cup is clean, it is clean all over."

Let your memory recall those great faith Scriptures mentioned earlier. Are we going to remove mountains and command sycamine trees? Are we going to be able to walk in divine health, cast out devils, heal the sick and raise the dead? We can! Because Jesus, in whom was truth made manifest, said, *"He that believeth on me, the works that I do shall he do also; and greater works than these shall he do . . . "* (John 14:12)

Faith . . . tremendous faith . . . is working in the Body of Christ today. We are looking forward to and claiming a manifestation of the promises of God. But we discover that at times we are disappointed, confused and frustrated in our efforts. Yet the day is only a sunrise away when we will not only see great miracles happening, but will be a part of it in a very active way. However, we must realize that all God's promises are conditional, especially for believers. *"Yet if any man suffer as a Christian, let him not be ashamed; but let him glorify God on this behalf. For the time is come that judgment must begin at the house of God: and if it first begin at us, what shall the end be of them that obey not the gospel of God? And if the righteous scarcely be saved, where shall the ungodly and the sinner appear? Wherefore let them that suffer according to the will of God commit the keeping of their souls to him in well-doing, as unto a faithful Creator."* (1 Pet. 4:16-19)

To those now, who are stepping out in faith with the Word of God to do as Jesus commanded and who do not see the manifestation for which they believed, I offer this explanation with the awareness that I, too, am seeing in part through a glass dimly:

The Sadducees knew the Scriptures, probably far better than did the apostles, but they were never able to do miracles, to heal, cast out devils or raise the dead, because they knew not the Word nor the power thereof. The Word is Christ. (John 1:14) And the power of the Scriptures is that which makes them Living Words: the Holy Spirit. (Acts 1:8; John 16:13) If we pray not in the Spirit, then we neither know how to ask nor what to ask and so we pray amiss. If we are praying from our heart's intent or from our intellect, there is no power in the Word except as it goes forth from our measure of faith and we wait upon the Lord.

Quoting words from the Bible doesn't give us magical power to transform material things or change circumstances.

I think a great many babes in Christ are being impressed that they can do just that, and when they don't see immediate results they become disillusioned and many fall away from the faith.

Reasonably, if we could just "speak the Word" and see immediate results, wouldn't the world be using the Word of God to further their own wayward and selfish ways? Could the Wisdom of God work at cross-purposes, knowing the evil intent of men's hearts?

There is no power in the Word of God unless the Holy Spirit gives the power! Therefore, it is always the wisdom of God which carries out the ultimate conclusion of a fervent prayer. It is "His Will" which is done on earth even as it is in Heaven. And the Word of God cannot be used as an incantation to bring about healings at our command, or cast out demons. Nor can the Word of God be used to increase a dollar offering to a hundred dollars. *"For our gospel came not unto you in word only, but also in power, and in the Holy Ghost, and in much assurance";* (1 Thess. 1:5) *"For the kingdom of God is not in word, but in power."* (1 Cor. 4:20)

Jesus said, *'But seek ye first the kingdom of God, and His righteousness; and all these things shall be added unto you."* (Matt. 6:33) *"But if I with the finger of God cast out devils, no doubt the kingdom of God is come upon you."* (Luke 11:20)

The kingdom of God is that realm wherein God Almighty is Omnipotent Sovereign Ruler. Man cannot enter that kingdom except by the New Birth, for nothing that he can attain by his mortal nature can gain his entrance into that divinely spiritual realm. Subjects of the kingdom of God must be wholly submissive and subservient to the King. In other words, the King reigns over His kingdom and no one can remain in that kingdom who is not surrendered unto Him. Only those who do the Will of the Father can enter in.

The initial entrance into the kingdom requires a commitment on our part to totally surrender our mortal desires to His divine and Holy Will and permit Him to be Master, Ruler of our lives. From that point on, as we learn obedience, we become more proficient in our status as residents of a Heavenly realm and appropriate the power given us through the Holy Spirit.

But where do most of us find ourselves? Honestly? Are we anchored completely within the kingdom of God or do we vacillate between His kingdom and that of the enemy? Jesus said, *"Every kingdom divided against itself is brought to desolation; and every city or house divided against itself shall not stand."* (Matt. 12:25) Power is not available to a person who serves two masters or divides his time between two kingdoms. Most of us fall into that category. We are not totally surrendered to Christ. There are still those vestiges of self we hold onto because of ego or pride or gluttony or fleshly desire or vanity or temper.

And so we pray. We patiently pray for ourselves and our loved one and for strangers afar off. We pray fervently the prayer of faith. We call for the elders and anoint with oil. We lay on hands. We confess our faults one to another. And, we pray, and ask, according to His will.

What is the will of God? Jesus said, *"And this is the will of him that sent me, that every one which seeth the Son, and believeth on him, may have everlasting life: and I will raise him up at the last day."* (John 6:40) Paul said, *"For this is the will of God, even your sanctification, that ye should abstain from fornication: That every one of you should know how to possess his vessel in sanctification and honor."* (1 Thess. 4:3-4)

Let us not, therefore, make absurd statements regarding the lack of God's response to our fervent prayer of faith, explaining the actions of God in such a way as to make Him look impotent or even worse, foolish. Such was the case, recently, when a Bible teacher was asked how a believer could die after having been prayed for, anointed, and hands laid on him. The answer was, "Oh, but he was healed!" The confused questioner responded, "But you don't understand. He died!" The teacher replied, "But for a believer, that is the ultimate healing. He goes to Heaven and has no more pain or sorrow. Oh, yes! He was completely healed of everything which ailed him!"

Perhaps you are thinking, "God, spare me that kind of healing, please!" No, death is not intended by God to be our ultimate healing. **The ultimate healing is the redemption of the mortal body so that there is no more death!**

We are being called as a body into deeper commitment unto holiness so that God can complete the Plan He has for us. But we have a long way to go, and such a short time to get there. There is so much more to accomplish for the kingdom. We need to be *"all with one accord"* (Acts 2:1) regarding divine health and healing, for the fields are white to harvest, even now, and the laborers are far too few!

In the chapters ahead we will consider physical health as it relates to the Word of God. May you find within these chapters the answer to your own health and healing.

2

"Lord, This World Makes Me Sick!"

I was suffering with acute ulcerative colitis, an illness which I'd had for some time. The condition steadily worsened, and although every mouthful of food caused me considerable pain, I persisted in prayer, believing that God would deliver me.

I'd been a champion worrier, one who did not realize that worry works against faith. I was like one who reads 18th century medical books for clues to exotic diseases, and then, in turn, diagnosed illnesses for family and friends. Twice each week, after viewing the television programs, Ben Casey and Dr. Kildare, my mind moved from calamity to crisis. And there I was, suffering with a real honest-to-goodness ailment which didn't go away at the end of the program. I was frightened! I'd finally reached the point in my affliction when all the alarm systems were sounding. I began to lose the mucous lining of the intestinal tract. I finally decided to see a doctor.

After listening to my list of symptoms, the doctor agreed

with my diagnosis. He prescribed several kinds of medicine to quiet the spasms of my poor convulsing stomach. Nothing helped. Neither the medicine; nor the vitamin injections or the baby food diet. Other prescriptions and drugs and different diets all failed. Weeks went by. I grew thin, pale and weak. My body was being drained of its vitality. I was beginning to fear that this ailment was the BIG ONE! "I am still very young," I thought, "and have so much to live for!"

Then, one day the Lord spoke to my heart and instructed me concerning what I had to do in order to be healed. It was so simple that I could hardly believe it. For the first time in months I had such a feeling of peace. I knew this would be the day of my deliverance!"

That afternoon a familiar car pulled into my driveway. I went outside with a calm and assurance I never had before. I walked over to the driver's side of the car. I smiled and said with a new authority, "Hello. I am glad to see you and hope that you will come inside and be our guest today. But I want you to know that, from this moment on, when you come to our house, it will be ONLY as a guest. This is our home. These are our children. The way we do things here is our business. The way we rear our children is our business. We can no longer permit you to interfere in our family affairs. If you will accept our relationship on those terms you are welcome to come here." — From that day on my colitis was healed and I've never again had a reoccurance.

I finally realized that medicine couldn't cure an affliction which was caused by inner turmoil and resentment. The cause of the physical condition had to be discovered and dealt with in a problem-solving manner.

I could have gone to doctors around the world and taken every kind of medicine and treatment known to man, but, until I got rid of the fear, anger and resentment, and the corresponding shame I felt for allowing such interference in my life, I would not be healed. The cause of the illness, which was an unconscious emotional conflict, had to be eliminated. When the conflict could no longer be contained in my person, it burst forth as an acute physical symptom. That is known as a "psychosomatic illness" . . . "psyche" is the Greek word for "soul" and "soma" is the body, thus indicating an illness affecting both the soul and the body.

The theory of psychosomatic illness is not new in the field of medicine. In fact, ancient and primitive medical practice had more regard for the effect of the soul upon the body than more modern practitioners, who consider only that which is visible under a microscope. German physicians were the first to use the term "psychosomatic" in professional writings as early as 1922. But the subject was not taken seriously until the early thirties when Dr. Helen Flanders Dunbar of *Columbia University College of Physicians and Surgeons* explored the depth of meaning in the term in her book, "EMOTIONS AND BODILY CHANGE."

A more recent outgrowth of the awareness of interrelationship between body and emotions has been the trend toward "holistic medicine," where there appears to be a tendency toward examing the cart to find out what ails the horse. One doctor stated that the condition of the body can effect the soul or spirit to ill health. Proper understanding of the sequential laws of the universe indicate, however, that the spiritual realm provides the pattern for the eventual manifestation of all matter.

Today, medical researchers are studying the correlations between spirit and body or emotions and body. Psychosomatic pain isn't imaginary, as any sufferer will tell you. It is real. And pain killers, or antibiotics, won't cure it. Even worse, the laying on of hands and prayer of the faithful won't, in most cases, alleviate the physical symptoms. I have seen people go to church altars week after week, seeking healing for the body, only to come away disappointed and sometimes lose faith in God because they felt He had not answered their prayers.

Our Father wants to answer every prayer which comes before His throne, but many times we, ourselves, hold back the answer by continuing in a state of dis-ease. Nor can we expect healing if we willfully sin. Twenty-five hundred years ago Hippocrates, the father of medicine, said, "In order to cure the human body, it is necessary to have a knowledge of the whole of things."

There are a multitude of variables which can adversely affect the body beside germs, viruses, antibodies and infections. Things such as the food we eat or don't eat, the chemicals we ingest, the pollution we breathe, the genetic factors of our familial line, the environment in which we are reared, the kind of job we have, the people we live with, and the type of personality we have.

All of these conditions may affect us; some of us are more

susceptible than others and each of us has our own way of coping with or overcoming the influences around us. But a proportionate number of ailing people are suffering from sicknesses which began in the soul as attitudes which are not in harmony with the nature of God.

We can't expect to have good health without a right relationship with God. It is impossible! All the nuances of uneasiness we experience before a God we may accept or deny are going to leave a mark upon us mentally, emotionally, physically, socially and occupationally. There is no escaping it. If we want physical and mental health, we must understand God's laws of the universe and the consequences we suffer for living in violation of them.

In Exodus 15:26 we read, *"If you will diligently hearken to the voice of the Lord thy God, and will do that which is right in His sight and will give ear to His commandments, and keep all His statutes, I will put none of these diseases upon thee, which I have brought upon the Egyptians; for I am the Lord that healeth thee."*

We have a reason for being on earth. Our personal causes, goals, aims and successes are nothing before the eternal purpose given to the soul of man at the beginning of time to return unto God with the self-conscious choice of surrendering all to Him. Along that route of religion (the word itself means: working our way back to God) we make many mistakes and have numerous victories and even a few triumphs. Through these endeavors at the personal level, we experience pleasure or pain, and by this, fashion the conscience of man.

The conscience is a part of the soul. Our inner witness. The "judge." When we act in opposition to the proddings of the conscience we experience pain. If we ignore this pain in the conscience or the soul, we eventually manifest a symbolic disorder at the physical level which we call "illness." If this illness manifests itself, it is a sign that we are still reacting to our conscience, even though at a hidden level. Some souls sink so deeply into sin and have ignored the conscience for so long that they no longer suffer the pangs of guilt and, consequently, there is no manifestation of any physical disorder.

Christians who lack understanding sometimes question the justice of God which permits blatant rebels to flaunt their sin in the face of the world without seeming to suffer the consequences. They fear that the infidels are "getting away with it." But they are not getting away with anything. Like Pharaoh, who also refused the cry of God, their hearts have been hardened and there is no longer an inner witness to help them respond to His voice.

Psychosomatic illnesses strike all of us. Seasonal colds, sinus infections, headaches, skin rashes, "female disorders," allergies and asthma are all warnings that we are out of fellowship with our Heavenly Father.

Some of the psychosomatic pains we feel haven't even developed into a physical affliction and yet the pain persists, causing apprehension in the patient and consternation in the doctor who deals only with the body. Some studies indicate that each of us has a physical place where we feel emotion, whether it be anger, joy, excitement or sadness. We may even have one place in the body which registers one kind of

emotion while another place in the body registers its opposite. We could interpret this as a kind of code being transmitted to us by our souls through our physical being.

This phenomena isn't a current juxtaposition. Historical
literature supported this correlation 4500 years ago when a
medical classic on psychosomatic illnesses was written in
China by Emperor Huang Ti. More recently, a survey of
163 patients in *John Hopkins Hospital* in Baltimore revealed
that 49% of the group studied had psychogenic disorders.
There were no physical findings to account for the symptoms
they suffered. An additional 27% had a combination of
physical and emotional disease. From the days of antiquity
to the present there is a wealth of material to suggest that
the concept of emotionally caused illnesses has occured to
those who seriously sought for an explanation of human
disease and misery. It was not considered equal to serious
study, however, until World War II, when the high incidence
of stress-related afflictions caused medical science to see,
with a new clarity, that everything we experience emotionally effects the physical.

Dr. Dunbar collected the results of her study and pub-
lished a thousand-page encyclopedia which listed psychosomatic interrelationship which has become a standard
medical reference book.

In the realm of religion, Martin Luther declared, in the
sixteenth century, that heavy thoughts brought on physical
maladies. He believed that when a soul was oppressed the
body reflected that state of mind in the form of some kind
of sickness. In those days it wasn't considered an oddity that

a person could die of a broken heart.

Physical illness can be a symptom of spiritual imbalance or disharmony with God. However, too many people choose to look for an explanation in other realms, believing sickness to be an accident or a contagion or just one of those hazards of life or an attack by Satan. Scientific studies would indicate, though, that most of these obvious explanations are a form of personal delusion. And, it is indicated that if we unquestioningly accept such a delusion, we won't be overcoming the problem, but will probably develop something more serious which will eventually force us to find the true origin of the malady.

The true origin of most of our afflictions appears to be spiritual rebellion, a condition which merits chastisement. If we come to understand why we have brought this chastisement upon ourselves, we will come out of the situation a better person. The Word says, *"My son, despise not the chastening of the Lord; neither be weary of his corrections; for whom the Lord loveth He correcteth: even as a father the son in whom he delighteth."* (Prov. 3:11)

How can we grow without correction? Left to our own devices, we quickly make excuses for ourselves or gradually fall away into deeper sin and rebellion. And that is not what we are called to do. We are called to walk in such a manner *"that ye may be blameless and harmless, the sons of God, without rebuke, in the midst of a crooked and perverse nation, among whom ye shine as lights in the world."* (Phil. 2:15)

That is our calling; especially now when we see the darkness closing in all around us, to be lights in the world, to set our light high on a mountain for all the world to see.

"And we know that all things work together for good to them that love God, to them who are called according to his purpose. For whom He did foreknow, he also did predestinate to be conformed to the image of his son, that he might be the first born among many brethren." (Rom. 8:28) Some of us live out our entire lives as Christians in name only, never receiving power to overcome and live victoriously. Now, as the new move of the Holy Spirit is filling the Church, so many are praying for power to be able to do great things for God while overlooking the admonition of our Lord that the cup must first be cleansed. Always, when we desire great things, sacrifices must be made. The kingdom of God will come to us, not in word only, but in power. First we must be made equal to that power. Jesus says to us yet today, *"I come that ye might have life and have it more abundantly."* (John 10:10 Paraphrased)

Abundant life would have to include health. Who can function to peak ability with chronic aches or acute pain? Who can be creative or inspirational with financial problems or marital discord? Who can give an effective testimony with carnal habits speaking louder than their words? We don't have to live that kind of witness. — If you have conditions in your life this *moment* which you know are not in alignment with the Word of God, pray for the wisdom to understand them so that you can be done with them. And then keep an open mind to be able to discern God's answer when it comes. If you presuppose your affliction is because *"the righteous suffer on earth but get their reward in heaven"* or that this is a Satanic attack, you won't be moving forward on your spiritual journey. More than likely, you have caused your affliction, somehow, either by something you have done or something you are refusing to do. Ask for the wisdom of God in the matter and it will come. Perhaps it will be in a still small voice, or maybe in a great shout. Perhaps it will be through some physical means such as a magazine article, or a book or a sermon, a song, a movie, a friend, or a dream. Whichever way it comes to you, it will be God answering your earnest prayer. Give Him the praise, honor and glory for He has, the very moment you cried out for wisdom, sent forth His ministering angel to bring you the answer you need to grow into the fullness of Christ.

Jesus is faithful to do that because He wants to see you healed more than you do. He suffered your affliction in all ways and has interceded for you before the Throne so that you would come to this place where you are right at this moment . . . seeking wisdom!

Paul taught, *"For though we walk in the flesh: (For the weapons of our warfare are not carnal, but mighty through God to the pulling down of strong holds;) Casting down imaginations, and every high thing that exalteth itself against the knowledge of God, and bringing into captivity every thought to the obedience of Christ; and having in a readiness to revenge all disobedience, when your obedience is fullfilled."* (2 Cor. 10:4-6)

We have weapons, spiritual weapons, to fight against those sorrows which inflict us with pain. These weapons given us by God are power from on High, the Holy Spirit, the interceding prayers of Jesus, the grace of our Father, and the victory Jesus won over powers, principalities and princes of darkness. These weapons of warfare will work to tear down the strongholds built up in our minds which have barricaded us from the love of God, WHEN OUR OBEDIENCE IS FULFILLED! This is the part we want to overlook: the obedience part; the part that says EVERY THOUGHT must be brought into the obedience of Christ!

Some of our thoughts have grown into attitudes which have put down deep roots into our subconscious minds. They grow there, like poisonous trees, bearing fruit which we unconsciously feed upon and offer to others. These bitter fruits make us sick, double us over in pain and yet we go back again and again for another bite because we fail or refuse to see the connection between the illness and what we are feeding upon. The power of God can destroy these poison trees and pull down the fortresses of negativity and delusion we have built around the forbidden orchard. Our Father wants to throw down every thought or attitude which has dominated us over and above the love of our creator. But we have to permit it. God will not force His way into our little created worlds, even if our creation is killing us! But if we allow Him, He will bring our thoughts into alignment with the thoughts of Christ! When we have allowed ourselves to surrender every thought unto Him, He stands ready to avenge Himself against the consequences of our disobedience!

Surrendering our thoughts unto Him means He will reveal us to ourselves. We will see ourselves as God sees us. Our weaknesses and shortcomings, our false attitudes and hypocrisies will stand out blatantly as God shines His Light into the

dark corners of our minds and hearts through the Holy Spirit,
the Spirit of Truth. That is what holds too many people back
from seeking the cause of their affliction. They really don't
want to know the truth about themselves. They say they
want the fullness of Christ but they don't want to accept the
fullness of themselves where they presently are. How can it
be that we can have our cake and eat it too? We have to give
up more and more of self in order to have more and more
of Him. John said, *"He must increase, but I must decrease."*
(John 3:30) John could say that about himself while Jesus
said of him that of man born of woman surely none was
greater than he!

We needn't fear having the truth of ourselves revealed
when it comes through the Holy Spirit. We can trust Him.
He will never hurt or humiliate us. His chastisement and
revelation will be given with such loving kindness and compassion that we can only rejoice that we are being delivered.
We *have* to see the truth of ourselves and our condition in
order to be delivered from it. That is the point of transformation.

The God of Israel says, *"Why should ye be stricken any
more? Ye will revolt more and more; the whole head is
sick, and the whole heart faint. From the sole of the foot
even unto the head there is no soundness in it; but wounds
and bruises and putrefying sores . . .* (Isa. 1:5-6) *"Wash you,
make you clean; put away the evil of your doing from before
mine eyes; cease to do evil; learn to do well; seek judgement,
relieve the oppressed, judge the fatherless, plead for the
widow. Come now, and let us reason together, saith the*

Lord; though your sins be as scarlet, they shall be as wool. If ye be willing and obedient, ye shall eat of the good of the land; but if ye refuse and rebel, ye shall be devoured with the sword: for the mouth of the Lord hath spoken it." (Isa. 1:16-20)

The Father says, *"Come, let us reason together."* To "reason" means to draw conclusions or inferences from facts or premises; to discuss or argue in a logical manner or to think out logically. He says, "Why should you be stricken anymore. Your whole body is sick, your relationship with the people around you is sick and your land is sick . . . what more do you need?" He wants you to cleanse yourself. How? By refraining from those things which are gainst God and start doing good works. By living according to His law of liberty and righteousness, with the reward of life eternal and overcoming the law of sin and death.

The first "good work" named for us to do is "seek judgment." Judgment means the act of deciding or passing decision on something or someone; judgment means good sense; discernment; understanding; opinion or notion formed by judging or considering; judgment means logic; the act of mental faculty by which man compares ideas and ascertains the relations of terms and propositions; a determination of the mind so formed, producing a proposition when expressed in words.

We are, therefore, asked to reason together with God to find out the logical, reasonable relationship between the calamities in our lives and the way we are living and believing. We are asked to use our minds and our powers of analysis,

deduction, observation, reasoning, experience, wisdom and
information to arrive at a logical conclusion which will
be proved out by the Word of God. I have met very few
people who are willing to do that. For some superstitious
reason, many Christians seem to be reluctant to use their
minds. They use limited knowledge sometimes of what
they believe the Scriptures teach but are reluctant to include
information which comes from other areas of life. They
classify scientific data and the results of medical research as
"worldly" and therefore of no consequence to the Christian
body. But we are in the world and the world affects us
whether we like it or not and God is in and through all
things. He can speak to us in any manner in which He
chooses. God can speak to us through science or medicine,
through education or through the arts. If our minds are
open to wisdom, God can speak to us anywhere at any time
through any means and He will give us the discernment . . .
if we are sincerely seeking His guidance . . . to know what is
false and what is true.

Logical reasoning affirms that in this cause-and-effect
world, nothing happens without impetus. Medical and
psychiatric research expose new evidence daily that what
and how we think has a direct bearing on the entire body.
Research has shown that our emotions can upset the en-
docrine system, alter the production of enzymes and hormones which must be maintained in intricate balance for
mental as well as physical health. There is accumulative
information indicating that certain types of personalities
are prone to certain kinds of diseases and those people can

be catalogued after a brief interview with a specialist. What does all this mean? Our minds DO affect the functioning of our bodies, and we will be able to be healed of certain conditions once we see the cause and are willing to allow the strongholds, which we have built over the years in our subconscious minds, to be torn down by the power of God Almighty.

If a person really wants to be delivered from an affliction and prays for an answer, it will come. But there are so many who do not want to know. Once you know that you are doing something which is causing the illness, you have the responsibility for it facing you. You either have to quit doing what is making you sick or you have to accept the fact that you'd rather be sick than change the attitudes or habits which are out of harmony with the will and wisdom of God. It is your prerogative. It isn't reasonable, but you can do it if you want to. You have the free will. Don't blame it on anyone else or expect other people to feel sorry for you. It was your choice and you took what you wanted. But if you want to put an end to it, ask for the reasonable explanation and the Lord will bring it to your mind and you will be delivered from that situation.

We have all heard that old but comforting adage that we are never given more than we are able to bear. It applies in this instance and is the reason why some people never get revelation knowledge about themselves. They are at the same place spiritually today as they were 20 or 30 years ago, when they first got saved. They knew, deep down inside, that there was more for them in the Christian life, but they didn't want to make the sacrifices necessary to have more. They have been satisfied with "just making it." But they wonder why it is they have hard times, sickness and emotional distress.

We've also heard the axiom, "the truth hurts." That is what keeps most of us from asking for revelation about ourselves. We don't really want to know the truth. But if you don't ever try to find the truth about yourself, you are never going to grow. How can you? You will persist in doing the same old thing the rest of your life. Be prepared to suffer the consequences for it because you most surely will. *"And they shall turn away their ears from the truth, and shall be turned unto fables."* (2 Tim. 4:3)

There are a lot of fables running rampant in the world today. Some of them are the little bedtime stories being embraced by a "liberated and modern society" which is intent . . . not upon growing in closer relationship with God . . . but on how to do your own thing without feeling guilty about it! This attitude has permeated the church who wants to be sophisticated and up-to-date. No wonder our health problems have been on the rise in the past twenty years and the cases of mental disorder have been multiplied faster than any other disease.

Psychologists who can make extra dollars writing for under-the-counter magazines would attempt to convince an insecure sex-and-youth oriented populace that, in order to have a healthy psyche, we must experience all aspects of life to the fullest without the burdening limitations which conscience would apply. Many of these counsellors

have gained national prominence as advisors for human behavior and have influenced thinking people at all levels of
our society but their teachings are Satanic lies and we must
have the spiritual discernment to see them as such in order to
maintain our balance in this crooked and perverse world.

Those Christians who seek help for problems from the
counsellors of the different schools of psychological theory,
sit in on encounter groups, sensitivity classes, engage in the
primal scream, sex therapy or whatever is currently in vogue
among the Godless, will discover that there is no help in these
areas and they will continue to suffer from the breaking of
God's law. And that is because God is still in control of this
universe. This is still His world.

I have observed so many "messed-up, freaked out" people
staggering out of the past decade who have tried to adapt
themselves to the humanistic religion of this age. For over
15 years I have worked with a large number of these people
and have studied their attitudes, reactions, responses and
watched the ultimate consequences of their philosophies.
It seems evident that psychology serves to intensify the
existing problems of most people rather than eliminate them.
Without God in the method of counselling and an understanding of the laws of the universe, there is neither help nor
healing!

*The body is afflicted because the soul is not in accord with
God.* And the soul is out of harmony because there is little
understanding of the nature of life. The spiritual side of life
is denied any importance whatever. How can healing take
place either temporarily or permanently in a body being

treated by a doctor or counsellor who would deny the very existence of a soul? And for that segment who claim a belief in the soul, how can they minister healing unless they acknowledge the Creator who made and animated that soul? Even the most sincere efforts are going to fall short of the mark. It's like a medical doctor trying to treat a severed arm by placing a band-aid on it. He may feel better for having done something, but the patient will die anyway!

A number of people suffered from fractured souls during the 1960's when "indepth therapy" was being attempted by anyone who had read a book on transactional analysis. Some zealous group leaders or members were too quick to zero in on another with unabashed honesty, pointing out their "hang-ups." A number of weak, inconfident, sensitive egos couldn't take it. Other group leaders believed that the way to overcome psychic disturbances was to trace them back to their origin and many probed beyond the barrier of the ego censor, resulting in some egos being scattered like broken strings of beads. There was neither compassion nor regard for what might be locked in the unconscious mind. Nor was there any sensitivity to enable the counsellor to discern how thin was the membrane between sanity and psychological collapse.

There are dark, mysterious secrets locked within our minds for which we, in order to maintain some semblance of balance in this world, have developed compensatory behavior. This compensatory behavior can be compared to ballast aboard a plane . . . it aids in keeping the balance until the proper cargo is loaded. Because we are not *filled* with the Holy Spirit, we easily can get out of balance. Unconsciously, we seem to sense that and we adapt certain behavior patterns which enable us to maintain a certain amount of balance until we come to fuller knowledge in Christ and are able to grow in the Lord.

Only God knows all that is hidden within our unconscious mind. Only He can see into those dark recesses and understand all that we have been through in our sojourn of life which has caused this compensatory behavior to form. He only can heal us utterly and completely.

These wells of recorded information hidden away within us have helped fashion what we are today. We don't remember many of these experiences. Some people remember less than others. They have taken every painful event and hidden the memory of it because they are too sensitive to live with the idea of pain. Even though the experience itself may be forgotten, we may react to the emotion these events stimulate every day of our lives.

It is then that we find ourselves acting out of compulsion; just like Paul we do that which we should not and that which we should do we do not. If we do not have an understanding of this compulsive behavior we find ourselves haunted by vague feelings of guilt, fear, tension and uneasiness. These disharmonious feelings trigger the production of enzymes or chemicals which can eventually break down our body's immune system and produce malfunctions of vital processes.

Or, we may develop systems of behavior to compensate for the uneasiness we feel and those actions may cause us further complications. Drinking, drugs, gambling, philandering, stealing, fighting, child or spouse abuse . . . all may originate from feelings of disassociation from God which the individual is unable to admit.

These acts are socially aggressive acts, some of them punishable by civil law. As long as we have some semblance of an ordered society someone will take care of the offenders. But not all people act out their aggressive feelings. Many go through a conflict between the animal instinct to strike out in self-preservation and the socially conformed method of suppression. And when a force that strong is being pushed down, where is it going to go? And who is going to mete out punishment to that one who entertained such murderous thoughts? The SELF will pass judgment and sentence oftentimes by afflicting the body!

That is another reason many people don't really want to be healed. Subconsciously, they are doing penance for the "bad" thoughts they held regarding certain people and situations. They are unconsciously expiating their guilt through suffering in the flesh. And no kind of healing . . . be it scientific or supernatural . . . will be able to take place when it is being applied only superficially to the flesh. An affliction also may be a balance stone for the conditions or people in their lives, which, very often, the ailing person finds impossible to tolerate. In a very real sense they are allowing the world to make them sick so they can continue living in it! And they are most likely making others in this world sick at the same time.

The colitis I had for such a long time is an example. It

helped me live with a domineering, critical, intimidating rela-
tive who made me very angry. Having been taught to show
respect for my elders, I didn't know how to be assertive. I
knew only how to act either passively or aggressively, a situation which provoked the strongest of aggressive responses in
my body. The instinct to strike out in self-defense produced
an oversupply of adrenalin. But I suppressed this primitive
urge and my own body was poisoned by the chemical which
was not burned in fight-or-flight energy. The anger made the
digestive acids of my stomach literally boil, resulting in gall . . .
(the word meaning "rancor and bitterness of spirit") . . .
pouring into my system.

When I got tired of being sick, I learned, with the help of
the Lord, that I had a better choice for dealing with my life
situation. I could act assertively and, thus, bring about a transforming experience in the lives of all of us. The greatest insight
I gained from that is that I have a responsibility to God to
allow no one to manage and dominate my life, but instead, to
let my life be under His control.

God knows where each of us is weak and what things are
needed for us to grow into the fullness of His image. We do
not achieve that divine goal by denying our sinful nature, but
by having it washed clean, redeemed and recreated by His
Spirit of love and the power of His Word.

Our growth is hindered if we permit someone to exert his
will over us. And, we are not being true to Him if we suppress
the call to follow Him.

Because of this experience with the colitis, the truth of
spiritual surrender has been written, indelibly, upon my

heart. Were all of this lesson inscribed in concrete language form, it would read, "If I am so anxious to get along with you that I allow you to exert your will over me, standing in the way of my fulfilling God's plan for my life, then I am selling my birthright for a mess of pottage . . . or for a peaceful home. You cannot hurt me more than you have already done!

'If I let you get away with exerting your will over me, I am standing in your way of coming to the Lord, because you may think that what you are doing is right. If I never stand up to you and establish that God is the only Master I am going to serve, how are you ever going to overcome taking charge of the lives of other people? Neither of us has the right to continue in this."

None of us can be expected to do that which is impossible to do. No one expects a three-month old infant to walk. We understand that there is a progression of growth that must take place and as it does, certain modes of behavior are adapted naturally. It is that way for a Christian, also. The whole Christian walk is an unfolding process somewhat like that of the unfolding of the petals of a rose. It is by taking one step at a time that we become the fullness of Christ. If we understand that and accept it, we can eliminate so much of the guilt which comes from knowing at some subliminal level of consciousness that we are not behaving as "good Christians."

I had three friends, all of whom epitomized our mental image of "good Christians." These three lovely, sweet-natured, spiritually conscientious women all died in their early forties!

One woman believed her marriage to be made in heaven and adored her husband as her eternal mate. She discovered, by accident, that he had engaged in a number of affairs throughout their marriage. She died suddenly and unexpectedly of a heart attack.

Another friend had a husband hurt and humiliate her to such an extent that she could neither forget nor forgive. She died of cancer of the liver.

The third young woman had a husband who beat her and her children. She cowered in fear before his angry abuse. She took his brutality without even a change in her sweet facial expression, declaring her love for him regardless of how he behaved. But she died a slow and agonizing death with a malignant brain tumor.

Researchers in psychosomatics have postulated that cancer is a form of suicide. For those who find life so unbearable and hopeless but have too much spiritual awareness to end their own lives, cancer is a method whereby they can unconsciously kill themselves without condemnation of God or family. Medical researchers have further found that cancer victims invariably have held the mental attitude for most of their lives that they are doomed to hopelessness and futility, never to realize the materialization of the heart's fondest dreams.

Of the three women above-mentioned, it is the last one whose memory I hold dear to my heart. We were the closest of spiritual friends and I took her illness as personally as I would have my own. We studied the Word together, prayed

for her healing. I drove her many miles to healing ministers
for annointing and laying on of hands. Many nights I prayed
through all the hours of darkness for her healing. I didn't
want her to die. I didn't want her to give up the fight. I
believed in God's ability to heal her but I didn't understand
why it didn't come.

She was a remarkable Christian. Her whole life from childhood on had been centered in the church and up until the
moment that she was unable to speak, she gave witness
to the glory of our Lord.

When she was in the cancer research hospital, she never
gave a thought to herself or her suffering and pain. Neither
did she allow the disfigurement of her illness to keep her
from being in the midst of people where she could serve the
Lord, even though she had possessed physical beauty and
charm before the ravages of cancer diminished her appearance. She had completely relinquished personal pride and
vanity. She went through the wards of the hospitals ministering to others who were in worse condition, giving testimony
to them of Jesus in her life and bringing hope and inspiration
to many who were frightened of the spectre of death hovering over them.

She wasn't afraid to die. She had absolute and complete
faith in the salvation bought for her through the blood of
Jesus Christ. Then why wasn't she healed in answer to our
prayers? Perhaps in the deepest part of herself where it
was hidden even from her own eyes, she didn't really want
to be. Perhaps she was more afraid to live in a world where
her sensitive spiritual nature was continually being con-

fronted with an animalistic brutality than she was to depart this world and enter into the next.

I like to think that Heaven is a place where we will "talk it over in the sweet bye and bye." I look forward to seeing my friend again, recounting the rainy days we spent at her house singing every song in the hymn book while she played the organ and we drank herb teas from tiny bone china cups.

I only wish she had known that her life needn't have been filled with rejection, hurt, abuse and fear. I wish we had been going to a real Bible-believing church where we would have been taught about the liberation of sin, sickness and death through the new birth in Christ. I wish we had known about the power of the Holy Spirit. Had that been the case, she would have been empowered to change all the circumstances in her life and be with us yet today. She could have had life and had it more abundantly. . . .

3

Does Sickness Come From God?

We Americans have become strong advocates of preventive medicine. Thousands of dollars are invested yearly in apparatus and equipment which temporarily ensures keeping the heart and pulmonary system functioning, the blood circulating, the muscles strong and the body limber. We jog, swim, skate, bicycle and hike. We go to spas, gyms, fat farms, health ranches and yoga ashrams, all in an effort to ward off bodily affliction. Although our billboards and glossy magazine ads would project us as ruddy-cheeked possessors of prolonged health, the *United Nations World Health Organization* states that we rank only twelfth in the world. Additionally, according to a survey done by the *Department of Health, Education and Welfare,* forty percent of all Americans suffer from one or more chronic diseases!

While Americans are pouring out hundreds of thousands of dollars annually for medical help to assist in healing a myriad of complaints, we continue to make ourselves sick by refusing to face the one common cause of our ailments.

The methods by which we achieve the singular end of illness are as varied as the personalities who succumb to the illness. The reasons we seek pain are complicated and often arcane. Generally, we can use the all-encompassing statement that our illnesses are caused by spiritual rebellion. Dissecting the other causes and categorizing them will, in the final analysis, place them under this one heading.

Physical and mental illnesses are often a reflection of our excesses and exaggerations. They indicate an imbalance somewhere in our entirety, whether it be at the mental level, or involving the emotions or perhaps a physical habit.

Illness and disease are many times meted to us by our conscience. This active element of judgment which is an essential part of the soul helps determine what is right and what is wrong for the person. The voice of the inner man warns us when there is trouble ahead. It is the conscience of man that tells him he deserves to be punished for rebelling against the laws of God. It is said that the soul chooses the *kind* of punishment from which the person will best learn.

None of our afflictions are one-dimensional; that is, affecting only the body. They are multi-dimensional and can be multi-faceted in their ability to teach us and help us open the inner man to greater strength than we have ever had before. Healing, therefore, involves the whole person, and if we are to be made whole we must begin to understand that which is involved in our sicknesses, by discovering the root cause. *"Fools because of their transgression, and because of their iniquities, are afflicted."* (Psa. 107:17)

Old Testament Israelites saw God as the giver of everything, good or bad. He was *Jehovah, Sovereign Ruler.* There was no other power. If they won a battle, Jehovah was rewarding them. If they lost, Jehovah was punishing them. When a child was born, it was a gift from God, but when a person died, it was interpreted that Jehovah had cut him off for some transgression. It was believed that sickness came from God. He was their Father and had the right to punish them for disobedience. Their responsibility was to grow under that chastisement and become more obedient to their Holy Father.

In my research into psychosomatic medicine I found that the ancient tradition of the Israelites may not have been mere superstition. The question is raised that, if it is a part of man's thinking or reasoning process which precipitates and preordains not only the fact of sickness but the special *kind* which is acquired, then would it not be necessary to understand the forces set into motion which could bring this sickness?

Since the reasoning faculty is of the soul and the conscience is part of that mental facility and the soul is the intermediary between God and mortal man, it may be that future scientific studies will have to entertain the possibility that the Scriptures were correct after all.

Currently, most medical men of the modern school concede that most illnesses seem to have originated in the psyche of the individual; however, they have not been able to determine why certain types of people succumb to certain kinds of ailments. More specifically, there are cancer-

type personalities, heart attack-type personalities, arthritis-
type personalities, high blood pressure-type personalities,
etc. Is there some hierarchal law of the spiritual realm which
subscribes a certain penalty for a particular sin?

If medical science would declare that such is the case,
would people thereafter take their afflictions more seriously
with regard to personal responsibility? Could such a declara-
tion prevent certain violations of spiritual laws? While all
this is only speculative at the present time, it is interesting
to note that the philosophy of today is completely different
from that of Biblical days.

Some people believe it is Satan who makes us ill. The
prescription for such an evil attack is to fight the enemy
with the Word of God and rebuke him in the name of Jesus.
These people probably recover at the same rate as those of
the world who lived in the time of Moses or Jeremiah. But
there was a big difference between them and the afflicted
of today. Ancient people had to search out their hearts to
find the iniquity which brought the affliction upon them,
confess it, and offer a sacrifice for reinstatement. They knew
the consequences for repeating the same mistake.

The person who thinks he is attacked by Satan might
lie in his bed feeling almost sanctified by his illness, thinking,
"The righteous must suffer." He groans upon his bed of
affliction, seeking pity because the enemy came against him
while assuring those around him that he never lost sight of
God's promises. He knows Jesus will deliver him. Regretably,
there are those who use sickness as a crutch and are "lame-
ducking it" throughout their Christian life when they could

be growing in glory and victory.

There are people who are ashamed of being sick when they know they shouldn't be. Their consciences are trying to tell them the cause of their illness but they don't want to hear it because the knowledge of it would necessitate some serious changes in their attitudes and emotions.

I know of a minister who teaches that if you are sick it is because of your unrighteousness. One day I saw this minister with puffy eyes, and dripping red nose, and with a voice hardly able to talk. I exclaimed, "What a terrible cold you have!" Quickly and indignantly the response was, "I do *not* have a cold! The Lord is giving me a new respiratory system!"

We see that one who walks in close communion with the Father, one who teaches and ministers to others, may find it even more difficult to admit having a physical problem. Perhaps that is why more ministers teach that sickness is a Satanic attack and not a chastisement from God. If he or she steps onto the platform on Sunday morning with a cast on their leg they have to be concerned that the congregation will be guessing which sin they've committed.

"Sin" means "missing the mark." It doesn't always mean robbing someone or committing adultery. Just missing the mark; not being right on target; being away from the center; out on the margin. Sin, then, doesn't always have to be doing something "bad." It could be not doing "good." Let us not "miss the mark" but live in the victory which Christ has provided for us through the Atonement.

Man is such a complicated being that, in the natural, it

seems impossible that he could ever be the fullness of Christ. Left to his own devices he would no sooner clean up one corner of his life than he would be confronted with a pile of debris in another corner. How glad we are that we do not accomplish our salvation through good works but through the blood of Jesus Christ. We *can* grow into the fullness of Christ and we should be consecrated to that inner work, but it is not to be undertaken in the way that one does psychotherapy, where the emphasis is on the problem and how to overcome it through understanding.

Digging up the past hurts and trying to analyze them does not cause one to grow and it may do more harm than good. Do you not agree that focusing one's attention upon Jesus and loving Him so much that the things of this world slip away is a much better way to deal with the contents of the subconscious mind? Our physical healing may take longer, but when it comes it will be a complete healing from the inside out, and the lesson which was intended by the affliction will have been learned.

The *caduceus* is the emblem of the medical profession as well as the insignia of *United States Medical Corps.* It is representative of the brasen serpent Moses had fashioned and placed upon the rod. When the children of Israel suffered from the bites of the serpents while in the wilderness, they were told that, in order to be healed, they should keep their eyes fixed upon the brasen serpent.

The Israelites were healed when they turned their attention away from the physical and focused upward, *"from whence cometh my help."* (Psa. 121:1b) They perceived the truth of divine life. When our minds are cleansed of the idea of sickness and both mind and spirit are brought into harmony with God, the body has to follow. Thus, healing is established.

God does not send "fiery serpents" to punish us but He permits them when man continues in his rebellious way. Our attitude of rebellion sets up currents of fiery bitterness which sting and bite not only the conscience but, in time, the body. To be healed, there must be a complete change of thought and a concentration, undivided, upon He who has given us all good and wonderful things.

When we turn our attention inward and allow our minds to dwell on the perfect ideal we have been given through the life of Jesus Christ, we bring about a harmonizing and uplifting process throughout our entire expression of life. Our vital energies will no longer be dissipated in the useless activities of worrying or complaining of ill health. Just as the loaves and fishes, all that the Lord has given us in life energy will be multiplied. With the help of our Creator we will use this creative substance to build a more abundant life.

God's will is for us to have wholeness . . . or holiness . . . of spirit, soul, mind and body. His will has never deviated from that perfect and absolute course. That is why He made available the Plan of Salvation through Christ Jesus. In order to bring us to a state of holiness, our Creator made every provision possible.

Yet, in spite of God's perfect love for us, we suffer and die daily. Good men and good women and innocent children die. Some turn away from the faith because they cannot reconcile the statistics of mortality with a God of Love. Could the church be largely responsible because they have not offered hope or explanation to man's dilemma? The two most important fields of thought pertaining to man, theology and psychology, are in warring camps, and, at best, are polite strangers to each other. Can we expect a greater apostasy than what is presently taking place in the world today?

The past thirty years have been an era of the greatest moral decline this nation has ever known. It coincides with the lopsided teaching of permissiveness propounded by an anemic church, frightened parents with too much bad advice and too little self-confidence, and a crop of teachers of the Huxlian "Brave New World" persuasion. The spirituality of Christian teachings has been obscured, to say the least.

Those who have maintained an attachment to Christian teachings have, for the most part, shared some of the neo-revelation of a God of Love. The chastising God of the Old Testament has been replaced with a "Father Knows Best" image who has a benign understanding of the human condition of weakness and sees us as well-meaning but rather foolish little creatures at whom He must wink and forgive.

From the bedrock of humanity has flowered the "New Age" teaching of the "Brotherhood of Man" – Humanism. This era has not yet come into full bloom. We have not acted upon all the insights we have gained during the past 15 years. Our present economical crisis is a grim reminder of this and yet the majority of people, in this country alone, are beligerantly resistant to the changes which must be made should any of us survive. Each group stubbornly clings to its pet indulgence while demanding the other to sacrifice and be understanding. But this stalemate has its dividends.

Christian leaders who don't want to call a spade a spade with the convicting power of Scriptural Word can stay clear of condemnation chortling and safely deliver a socio-political message without ever mentioning that banned topic: Sin! But establishing programs which attempt to distribute physical necessities more evenly throughout society is not getting to the core of the problem, which is the loss of inner stability.

It is this loss of inner stability which can most likely be traced as the precipitator of other human ills, nationally as well as personally.

Claude Bernard, foremost French physiologist of his day, said of stability: "It is the fixity of the 'inner condition' which is the condition of free and independent life, and all the mechanisms, however varied they may be, have only one object: that of preserving constant the conditions of life in the internal environment."

Paul exhorted, *"Therefore, brethren, stand fast, and hold the traditions which ye have been taught, whether by word, or our epistle."* (2 Thess. 2:15) *". . . be ye stedfast, unmoveable, always abounding in the work of the Lord, forasmuch as ye know that your labour is not in vain in the Lord."* (1 Cor. 15:58)

Leon Fredericq said, "The living being is an agency of such a sort that each disturbing influence induces by itself the calling forth of compensatory activity to neutralize or repair that activity. The higher in the scale of living beings the more complicated do these regulatory agencies become. They tend to free the organism completely from the unfavorable influences and changes occurring in the environment."

These three gifted men, Bernard, the Apostle Paul, and Fredericq, observing the human condition and approaching it from different avenues, agree on one single solution: innter stability . . . or *"the peace of God, which passeth all understanding."* (Phil. 4:7a)

If we examine the human nervous sytem we note that it is divided into two parts: the central nervous system and the peripheral nervous system; simply, one part acting outwardly and affecting the world around it and the other acting inwardly and helping to preserve a constant and steady condition of the body. E. Stanley Jones interpreted this as reflecting the necessity of maintaining a"strength" which keep us inwardly steady and a "power" that can change the outer conditions in our lives, and if not change them, empower us to adaptation.

The wisest man in the world, Solomon, obviously understood the necessity of maintaining such inner balance or stability in order to withstand the inconsistencies of the world about us. And because he *"built the house of the Lord and his own house,"* (1 Kings 9:15) he knew far better than anyone the essential requisite in spiritual power.

And so Solomon, the man of peace, built the temple in Jerusalem, the habitation of peace, and in the building of this temple he laid the plans for the building of "our" temples, the body incorruptible!

Solomon's temple is a type of our completed being in Christ. Studying the components of the temple brings tremendous insight into what God has planned for us and what requirements we will have to meet to begin our temple. The first requirement is inner peace or stability!

The two pillars placed in front of the temple were the first thing the pilgrim would observe. Fifty feet high and overlaid with brass, they reflected the rising sun to all the inhabitants of Jerusalem each morning. Those pillars did not support any of the architecture of the temple so the purpose would have to be symbolic.

Solomon named the two pillars after two men: Jachin, on the right hand, and Boaz on the left. Jachin means *uprightness* and *strength.* Boaz means *in power.* Symbolically, the right side represents giving from within; the left side represents receiving from without. The right side deals with an inner state of consciousness and the left deals with outer conditions.

In making the temple of Solomon a representation to all future generations of what we shall become in our perfected state, the Lord reminds us that it takes strength to maintain our equilibrium no matter what is going on about us. And only the power indued to us from on high can change our environment or circumstances for the better.

When we act in opposition to the laws which have been impersonally established, we bring about a state of instability, not only to ourselves, but to this world. When enough people act out of common instability, the results are paramount. Our country alone had 80,000 teenage suicide attempts in one year. How much more unstable does our world have to become before we collectively seek the solution?

Will the answer be what most people are fearing . . . some calamity which will chasten the people to such an extent that they will bow their knees and turn to God? Amazingly, among those apocalyptic thinkers is a fair number who do not entertain any other Christian ideas. The theme of "Divine Judgement and the Ultimate Punishment" seems to be written on the hearts of all mankind.

What is it in man that he expects, even waits for, punishment for his wrong doing? Is it because in the rearing of our children we have told them, by example, that we have set certain limitations upon them, not out of pernicious intent, but rather because we could see the inherent dangers ahead for them and wish to spare them?

An obedient child will follow rules and avoid a lot of hurt and pain. But the child who doesn't obey is sure to be hurt time and time again, either by his actions or by the parent who discovers his disobedience and metes out his deserved punishment. The child who isn't chastised will probably not be hindered in his rebellious actions.

Last summer there was a sad incident involving four young boys who climbed over the fence around a public pool in the middle of the night to go swimming. All drowned. The pool was drained and no other children in that neighborhood will be able to swim there again. People asked, "Where were the parents of the pre-teen boys who were out in the middle of the night?" ". . . *whom the Lord loveth, he chasteneth, . . . "* (Heb. 12:6) Could it be that, "whom the parent loves, he also chastises?"

To chastise means to inflict suffering upon for purposes of moral improvement; discipline or subdue, as by adversity; to restrain, moderate or temper; make chaste in style; to castigate, which means to punish in order to make pure or correct." Chastisement, therefore, is a positive force, put into action by love with regard for our ultimate position.

Why, then, do we doubt that a loving Father God would chastise His children? In times past it was not a difficult concept to accept because fathers fulfilled their rightful roles as spiritual leaders of the family. Versed in Scripture, fathers then acted out the Biblical role assigned to them. They were to teach of God's way to wife and children. The rebuking rod had its place in those homes. In today's society there are many homes which are devoid of any rebuking rod.

It is childish to expect a father to pour out blessings . . . *"whatsoever ye shall ask in prayer,"* (Matt. 21:22) . . . with no conditions applied while we continue to serve selfish purposes. The Old Testament Jehovah, Lord most vehement, spoke emphatically, *"And thou shalt not go aside from any of the words which I command thee this day, to the right hand, or to the left, to go after other gods to serve them. But it shall come to pass, if thou wilt not hearken unto the voice of the Lord thy God, to observe to do all His commandments and His statutes which I command thee this day; that all these curses shall come upon thee, and over-*

take thee . . . " (Deut. 28:14-15)

Our Heavenly Father is a God of mercy, love, forgiveness and patience. But if we have chosen, by the exercise of our free will, to live in disobedience and rebellion to Him, can we blame Him for "allowing" justice to prevail? *"Though He were a Son, yet learned he obedience by the things which He suffered; And being made perfect, he became the author of eternal salvation unto all them that obey him . . . "* (Heb. 5:8-9)

Too long we have viewed God through a pin-hole, seeing only one tiny facet of His Nature and denying the whole. This kind of fragmented thinking reminds us of the parable of the blind men who tried to describe the whole elephant by the single part of the animal they were touching. Yes, God is the personification of love and mercy; He is the Creator but He is also the Destroyer! *"The Lord shall send upon thee cursing, vexation, and rebuke, in all that thou settest thine hand unto for to do, until thou be destroyed, and until thou perish quickly; because of the wickedness of thy doings, whereby thou hast forsaken me."* (Deut. 28:20)

Can any of us deny that it is a terrible thing to fall into the hands of the living God? Can you not examine your life and say that you, because of your spiritual rebellion, have seen the fury of God? *"And after all that is come upon us for our evil deeds, and for our great trespass, seeing that thou our God hast punished us less than our iniquities deserve, and hast given us such deliverance as this . . . "* (Ezra 9:13) *"For our light affliction, which is but for a moment, worketh for us a far more exceeding and eternal weight of glory . . . "*

(2 Cor. 4:17)

To speak of a chastising God provokes considerable discussion concerning the Law versus Grace. The argument is: "If we are under Grace, then the Law is abolished." Yet Jesus said He came not to abolish the law but to fulfill it. Some argue, "We are under a new covenant." But didn't Jesus say, *"Till heaven and earth pass, one jot or one tittle shall in no wise pass from the law, till all be fulfilled."* (Matt. 5:18) The argument continues, "Jesus finished all the work which was needed to be done to unite mankind with the Father." Jesus said, *"Be ye therefore perfect, even as your Father which is in heaven is perfect."* (Matt. 5:48) Their response, "We can have no righteousness other than the righteousness of Jesus who has joined us to Himself even as He is joined to the Father." But didn't Jesus say that unless our righteousness exceeded the righteousness of the scribes and Pharisees we could in no case enter into the kingdom of Heaven? Jesus did not do away with the Law, but rather intensified it! He took that Law which was burdensome to its adherents in outward rituals and practices and applied it to inward attitudes of the heart and prejudices of the mind.

Paul answered the Christians in Rome, "Are we doing away with the Law? God forbid! We are establishing it!" (Rom. 3:31 Paraphrased) We walk in the Spirit according to the Law and fulfill the requirements of holiness by the exercising of inner strength which comes from our Lord. With this consecration to holiness (we shall not see the completion of it in this flesh) comes the proportionate power from on high to act in the Name of Jesus and have dominion over the forces about us. *"Be not deceived; God is not mocked: for whatsoever a man soweth, that shall he also reap. For he that soweth to his flesh shall of the flesh reap corruption; but he that soweth to the Spirit shall of the Spirit reap life everlasting."* (Gal. 6:7-8)

When Paul complained of the law, he spoke as a Jew who had lived some 30 to 40 years carrying out the endless disciplines which were necessary to remain a good Jew. To neglect one of these little ordinances was to have broken all the Law. Under such conditions there was no way to have inner peace or stability. It must have been much like waiting under the sword of Damocles. It is understandable that Paul would disdain that Law and rejoice in the new freedom of the Law Jesus espoused, which is known as "sowing and reaping" — the *Divine Law of Retribution and Compensation.* It is believed by many in the Christian world to be the underwriter of the tribulations we suffer.

Emerson said, "Cause and effect, means and ends, seed and fruit, cannot be severed; for the effect already blooms in the cause, and the end pre-exists in the means, the fruit in the seed."

The process of sowing and reaping or retribution and compensation is in operation at all times within the individual life, group life, national and planetary life as we individually and collectively strive to establish balance and harmony. This Law, which is the major domo from which all other laws extend, is working simultaneously within us and around us, at every level of awareness and expression known to creation. ALL things will be brought to submission unto God Almighty!

Was it this Law of which David spoke when he said that the Law of the Lord is perfect, that it converts the soul? To meditate upon the *Law of Retribution and Compensation* would indeed make changes in us for from that meditation would come the enlightening revelation of what we, individually, have put into effect in our lives. We have the power to ordain what our future shall be by making the right choices *in accordance with the will of God.* There is no chance, no accident, no injustice, no persecution. We each receive just chastisement *by the law* and the deserved recompense. Even Paul's persecution after his conversion . . . wasn't it exactly what he had done to other Christians before his conversion? Of course, he was forgiven. But who could stop what he had put into motion such a short time before? *There are people who think they are being attacked by Satan but are only reaping what they have sown in an earlier planting.* And the impetus which began their difficulty is no different from what you and I suffer, all of which will be covered in the chapters ahead. 1 John 5:18 says, *"he that is begotten of God keepeth himself, and that wicked one toucheth him not."*

Another Scripture says, *"But if ye be led of the Spirit, ye are not under the law."* (Gal. 5:18) Consider that Christ is *over* that law and if we be led of the Spirit, we are over the law with Him for He has lifted us up to sit with Him in high places. This is the amazing promise of our salvation, one which no other religion or its founder can offer. For Christ alone has the power of God and He has empowered us through the Holy Spirit that we can follow Him and go where

He has gone! His blood can cleanse us from iniquity, His Word can wash us clean, His power can break the bondage which holds us.

"Blessed is the man that walketh not in the counsel of the ungodly, nor standeth in the way of sinners, nor sitteth in the seat of the scornful. But his delight is in the law of the Lord; and in his law doth he meditate day and night. And he shall be like a tree planted by the rivers of water, that bringeth forth his fruit in his season; his leaf also shall not wither; and whatsoever he doeth shall prosper." (Psa. 1:1-3)

Whatever we have set into motion by the attitudes, actions. convictions and emotions within us will come upon us in due season. And when it does, resist it not. Agree with it when it comes to you because it is yours; you have made it and you must learn by receiving what you have given out to others. If you agree with it, recognize it for what it is and why it is come upon you, confess it and ask for God's mercy and the affliction will leave you.

When we are visited with the refiner's fire and fuller's soap, let us not carry on like big crybabies. *". . . Resist not evil . . . "* (Matt. 5:39) *"Agree with thine adversary quickly, whiles thou art in the way with him; lest at any time the adversary deliver thee to the judge, and the judge deliver thee to the officer, and thou be cast into prison. Verily I say unto thee, Thou shalt by no means come out thence, till thou hast paid the uttermost farthing."* (Matt. 5:25-26)

The soul of man is striving constantly to maintain a delicate balance between the forces of God and the forces of nature. We can heal and be healed only when we are willing to establish a consistent balance of harmony between the body, mind, soul and spirit and the Spirit of God.

If we are not willing to establish such harmony and inner stability, then we must accept the truth that we have, with full knowledge, chosen to live in disobedience, and incur the chastisement of the Father. No excuses, no self-pity. No long discourses about our doctor's reports, or lab results. Our bodies, or our circumstances or our finances are ailing because at some point we have chosen to live in rebellion at some level of our being. *"Be not wise in thine own eyes: fear the Lord, and depart from evil. It shall be health to thy navel, and marrow to thy bones."* (Prov. 3:7-8)

The Lord will warn us consistently when we veer off the right path. He will speak to us through His Word and through His servants. If we ignore the warnings we will suffer the consequences of our unrighteous living.

It is our Father's desire to bring us into obedience. As the indwelling Spirit of God fills us more completely, and we come to greater and greater understanding of His tremendous love for us, we experience a deep longing which nothing else can fill. That longing is to be fully in His presence; to be fully possessed by Him and bathed in His glory. Then it is no longer a struggle to surrender our will to His. It becomes a willing choice.

The natural man does not long for things of the Spirit. They mean nothing to him. He cannot comprehend them. Indeed, they are foolishness. It is only as he learns, through the painful lessons of the flesh, that the world of sense and matter is laden with frustration, disappointment, and false allure that his soul is stirred by the Holy Spirit. When all of this world has been tried and found wanting, when one road after another leads only to a dead end, when the pain of utter hopelessness overcomes the soul till it appears there is no light left in the world, then does the soul cry out, "God! Have mercy!"

Pain, like chastisement, can be a positive force. Where you stand at the present, it may not seem to be so, but forebear! The work is not yet finished for pain, as nothing else, purifies us for the greater work ahead! No religious service, love-outreach or stringent discipline can do for the soul what the process of pain can do!

Pain can burn away the veil which separates the human self from the immortal soul. Dr. Richard Maurice Bucke, author of the classic "COSMIC CONSCIOUSNESS" said, "I have learned the grand lesson, that suffering is the price which must be paid for all that is worth having; that in some mysterious way we are refined and sensitized . . . so that we are made susceptible to nature's higher and finer influences."

By itself, however, pain does not make saints or gods of any of us. It is not the mere occasion of suffering which elevates us spiritually . . . it is the ability to be able to transmute that pain into a tangible elixir which the soul can digest: wisdom!

The period of renunciation and transmutation which follows the cycle of pain and suffering is probably the singularly most important phase of earth man's life. It is usually not just one period during the span of a lifetime but rather may come several times until we learn the lesson of sacrifice.

"I beseech you therefore, brethren, by the mercies of God, that ye present your bodies a living sacrifice, holy, acceptable unto God, which is your reasonable service." (Rom. 12:1).

Sacrificial periods come regularly throughout our lives. Each cycle requires a surrendering of self and if the sacrifice is made willingly, there is little pain involved. But if we refuse to relinquish that which was never ours to begin with; if we persist in clutching to ourselves that which is required to lay upon the altar, the burden of debt becomes greater for the next cycle. Consequently, the pain at relinquishing becomes stronger.

Those who are open to receive the promptings of the soul are aware of what is required during the period of sacrifice, but man . . . bound by his carnal nature, does not make a willing pilgrimage to offer a sacrifice of self or the material gains of this world.

Straining to maintain that which he feels is slipping away increases his pain. This may continue for weeks, for days or even for years until he senses his physical strength waning and he can no longer maintain his hold upon the things of this world. When that moment comes, there is a feeling of resignation, surrender. What does it matter any more, he may decide and his fingers are then pried loose from that which he called "mine."

There is then a feeling of freedom which follows; sweet release; chains of bondage snapping loose on the heart. We feel a fresh breeze moving within us, a sweet odour, a warmth and the windows of our souls are then thrown open to let in the Light. The night is over and we have survived! Joy cometh in the morning! And it is now a pleasure to say with all sincerity and trust, "Father, Thy will be done, on earth, as it is in Heaven!"

4

You Are What You Think!

Remember the nursery rhyme about the little girl with the curl in the middle of the forehead? When she was good she was very, very good but when she was bad, she was horrid! Does she remind you of anyone you know?

When I was younger and had a more limited understanding I thought I had a split personality because I was like the girl in the poem. Very good sometimes and very horrid. When I was in one of my stormy moods I saw everything inside out and upside down. White was black and black was white. And I hated myself! When I was good, I was inspired and inspiring, magnanimous, gracious, patient, loving and generous . . . the virtues of a saint fairly radiated from me. How the "other me" caused me grief and guilt! I could see that these two faces were complete opposites and, naturally, I wanted to identify with the good person.

At that time, this *duality* was a mystery to me. I didn't know then that we all have it; that it is one of the consequences of Adam and Eve's rebellion, and gives evidence that the inner man and outer man struggle for dominance in this body of clay. Paul described this very conflict even after his dramatic conversion and complete dedication to Christ! The fact is we are dual in nature and double-minded and for most of our lives, the two sides of our nature are trying to pull the spirit-man in two opposing directions.

To illustrate this, let us imagine a man riding in a buggy drawn by two horses; a white one on the right and a black one on the left. The white horse is trying to pull the buggy one way while the black horse is intent upon going in the opposite direction. Obviously, the man is going to have to struggle to gain control over the horses. He'll have to get them going in the same direction or the buggy will be over-turned.

More explicitly, the man represents the human spirit, and the horses represent the dual natures of the soul which are responding to opposing stimuli and the buggy represents the mortal body.

The spirit-man is the real self; the body is neutral, merely following whichever way it is lead by the stronger force of the soul. And the soul, until that time of awakening in Christ, is divided between the force of heaven and the near-irresistible drawing of the forces of earth.

Once I recognized the duality of my nature, I was deter-mined that I would drive the divided factions of my soul and maintain a tight rein over them so that I would be able to move forward in my journey of life. I could see that allowing the "horses" to do their own thing kept me from obtaining true victory in the Christian walk. It was constantly one step forward and a dozen backwards. So I began an introspective study of myself, determining which aspects I wanted to develop and enlarge upon and which aspects needed to be eliminated. *"Look carefully then how you walk, not as unwise men but as wise, making the most of the time, because the days are evil. Therefore do not be foolish, but understand what the will of the Lord is."* (Eph. 5:15-17 R.S.V.)

I discovered that the dark side of me (the natural man) gained opportunity for dominance when I was tired, when I didn't feel up to par, when I dieted, when I didn't get enough sleep, and when I ate sweets. But the natural man didn't stand a chance for expression when I was well-rested, ate a balanced diet, when I took time out from the obligations of motherhood and housekeeping to read my Bible, when I felt I looked attractive, when I got away from the house to fellowship with other Christians and when I was involved in charity or something creative.

When the inner man was dominant, I felt good about myself and about everyone around me. I had a good relationship with people, with myself and with my Lord. But when the outer man was dominant, I was out of harmony with the world. After such a discovery, wouldn't it make sense, thereafter, to do what was necessary to allow the inner-man to have dominant expression in my life? It wouldn't make sense to continue doing those things which burdened me with guilt and hindered my prayer life. *"Behold, we put bits in the horses mouths, that they may obey us; and we turn about their whole body."* (James 3:3)

Every infraction of Divine Law brings sorrow and pain. If

we always would abide in the fullness of His law of love we wouldn't have need of either. No matter how much we might want to reject the idea that we have brought our painful experiences upon ourselves, the truth keeps jumping at us. We are not what God intended us to be, nor are we what we think ourselves to be. There is improvement yet to be made for which *we* must take the responsibility.

Henry Thoreau said, "If by patience, if by watching, I can secure one new ray of light, can feel myself elevated . . . shall I not watch ever?" How often I have viewed the six o'clock evening news with a grieving heart, as I am reminded that in 2000 years the human race has advanced so little toward the lessons Jesus taught. It isn't wanton defiance on our part that we continue to crucify Him. It is lack of understanding of our own responsibility in the matter. *"Wherefore, my beloved, as ye have always obeyed, not as in my presence only, but now much more in my absence, work out your own salvation with fear and trembling. For it is God which worketh in you both to will and to do of his good pleasure."* (Phil. 2:12-13)

It is only in those who have been touched by God, those who have felt the reality of His Presence, that such a work of conversion or soul-changing can begin. Whether that change is instigated because we seek healing of the body, relief of the conscience, rectification of personal relationships or consecration of our religious intent, we begin with the conscious choice of controlling the double factions of the soul. *"Wherewithal shall a young man cleanse his way? By taking heed thereto according to thy word."* (Psa. 119:9)

Many times, Jesus admonishes us to "take heed." *"Take heed therefore unto yourselves and to all the flock . . . "* (Acts 20:28a)

Webster's Dictionary defines the word *heed* as: "To listen to with care; to take notice of; to attend to or give attention."

We undertake, then, to give attention to or listen to the *self* — the real person within — to take notice of the self and its needs, attitudes, convictions and pains. It involves looking into the self, objectively, and seeing our innermost being as it really is. The answers we seek to those age-old questions "Who am I? What am I? Why am I here? Where am I going?" are the beginning of spiritual awakening. *"Wherefore he saith, Awake thou that sleepest, and arise from the dead, and Christ shall give thee light."* (Eph. 5:14)

But what, exactly, is the "self"? We can simplify it by saying it is the "I am"; the aggregate of spirit, soul and body. We might say that it is man's consciousness with its triplicity, including also, the superconsciousness and the subconsciousness. Yet we must include what we are physically, for does not the physical also play a part in the total person? Some say "the self" incorporates every experience we have ever had, every person we have had contact with and our response to both.

Eastern tradition holds that there are two selves; the higher and the lower self . . . twins . . . vying for position; the watcher and the doer; the master and the apprentice; the guide and the traveller; the lord and the servant.

Judaism uses the symbology of Ishmael and Isaac, the bond and the free, to express the same idea. Jesus told the parable of the prodigal and the faithful sons.

Whatever symbology we use to convey the idea of self-hood, the predominant theme remains, that there is that one part of us which is the wiser and which also seeks to do the will of the Father, and that one part of us which defies that which is good and right and is part of our Adamic nature. Our wiser part impresses us with the guardian benevolence which we often ascribe in our dreams as an angel.

Becoming aware of self can be a lifetime vocation, for, once begun, the ego senses its ultimate slaying and fights for a firmer hold. Yet, persisting in understanding the complexity of our nature has the highest reward . . . the illuminating presence of He who made us in His image, flooding our inner being with His glorious light. *"That he would grant you, according to the riches of his glory, to be strengthened with might by His Spirit in the inner man; . . . "* (Eph. 3:16) It is more than a thousand times worth the struggles for even a brief moment of that glory.

We can begin this occupation by studying the body; its cravings, desires and demand for attention which tries to draw us away from Him. Then, as we turn the mind away from the body to study the response of the senses and how they try to entice and delude us, we realize further how the natural man works at cross-purposes against the inner man. We can then move deeper inward to the font of our emotions where we will realize that sometimes we get conflicting signals, that the emotional nature is harder to train than the mind, that the emotions operate against the will and often presage conditions in the body.

From the emotions, we move our attention to the process of thinking and begin to learn how, dispassionately, to view our thoughts. We needn't fear the contents of the mind which rise unbidden from the wells of the unconscious, but we should be aware which thoughts belong to us and which ones have been broadcast to us by the prince of the power of the air. Over this we must exercise the authority of our will. This is the area where the major battle between light and darkness takes place and Satan tries, in every way possible, to keep us from discovering our spiritual minds. If the contents of our thoughts frighten us enough, the carnal mind is secure in having control of both the ego and the will. This can keep us from overcoming the limitations of bondage. *"To set the mind on the flesh is death, but to set the mind on the Spirit is life and peace. For the mind that is set on the flesh is hostile to God; it does not submit to God's law, indeed it cannot; and those who are in the flesh cannot please God."* Rom. 8:5-8 Paraphrased)

All the influences we receive from the carnal man are part of the delusion in which we have been held in bondage. But now, the "Body of Christ" is in the process of breaking free. It requires an urgent and stringent discipline on our part, but those who have the Spirit of God indwelling them know that, through Him, we can do it. *"Train yourselves in godliness; for while bodily training is of some value, godliness is of value in every way, as it holds promise for the present life and also for the life to come. The saying is sure and worthy of full acceptance. For to this end we toil and strive, because we have our hope set on the living God, who is the Savior of all men, especially of those who believe."* (1 Tim. 4:7b-10 R.S.V.)

When we endeavor, then, to train ourselves in godliness, the way is prepared for us to enter into the Kingdom of God within where we begin to worship Him in Spirit and in truth. (John 4:23) For it is not until then that we can come close to that altar, not built with hands, where the Pillar of Shekinah . . . the Divine Fire . . . abides. And in that moment, we will know, with a surity, the real self, created in the Image and Likeness of God. We will willingly surrender all to, *"Put off your old nature which belongs to your former manner of life and is corrupt through deceitful lusts, and be renewed in the spirit of your minds, and put on the new nature, created after the likeness of God in true righteousness and holiness."* (Eph. 4:22-24 R.S.V.)

There is no freedom outside of Christ. People all across this land are espousing movements to declare their "liberation" but they won't find it until they become liberated in Christ. Those who answer that higher calling, who have given up everything which has held them in bondage to the flesh, willingly cut the ties which bind the soul to the personality with its self-deception. Others, sensing the sacrifices they must make, resist this "dying to self" because they fear losing something of intrinsic value. But is this true? "It is impossible," some say, "to find that pearl of great price, unless everything we possess is sold." We have been taught, *"Blessed are the poor in spirit: for theirs is the kingdom of heaven."* (Matt. 5:3).

This spiritual poverty or humility is the result of allowing the Holy Spirit to work within us instead of permitting our personal egos to dominate our will.

The kingdom of heaven is a state of consciousness in which the soul and the body are in harmony with God. Jesus said . . . *"The kingdom of God cometh not with observation: Neither shall they say, Lo here! or, lo there! for, behold, the kingdom of God is within you."* (Luke 17:20b-21) How many of us claim a kingdom of heaven within when we are haunted by thoughts which plague us with guilt, shame, resentment, and uneasiness?

" . . . and I will take the stony heart out of your flesh, and will give you a heart of flesh. And I will put my spirit within you, and cause you to walk in my statutes, and ye shall keep my judgments, and do them. And ye shall dwell in the land that I gave to your fathers; and ye shall be my people, and I will be your God. But as for them whose heart walketh after the heart of their detestable things and their abominations, I will recompense their way upon their own heads, saith the Lord God." (Ezek. 36:26-28; 11:21)

It is out of the heart of man that proceeds all issues of life. Once I worked for a man who tried to be very gruff and cold, but one could see that from his heart he wasn't like that at all. He was a very warm and kindly man but undoubtedly thought that if his employees didn't fear him, they wouldn't work as well for him. So he assumed a "tough" role. One day he stomped and barked at his salesmen for over an hour, obviously believing this was the best way to inspire them to work harder. After the meeting, I stuck my head in his office and teasingly told him, "Why do you act like a 'cross bear'? We all know you are a good man and have chosen the best people you could find to work for you. Don't you trust your judgement anymore?" For a moment, he was startled. No one had ever before dared to be that personal with him. His face turned bright red. Then he quickly recovered and "harumphed" while his blue eyes twinkled. He couldn't hide what he really was in his heart. At Christmas time that year, he gave me a double bonus.

The dual natures of the soul, inclining us either toward the heavenly realm of God or the earthly realm of self, contain the potentiality of all the best or the worst of which man is capable. The soul touches both the *inner realm* of Spirit where it receives direct revelation from the Spirit of God, and the *external realm* where it is impressed by the enamoring temporal enticements of the physical.

As the soul is torn between the two extremes of the peaceful sanctuary of the Spirit and the chaotic conditions of the personality, it learns . . . oftimes, simply through the process of trial and error . . . to bring all the conditions of experience under the influence of the divine consciousness of the indwelling Spirit. It is then that we establish harmony with our Father God and discover that we are beyond the confusion of the outer world. We are in it but not of it. We shall be maintaining peace in the center of chaos. We shall be the calm in the eye of the hurricane.

The most unhappy, hard-to-live-with people in the world are those who do not have a glimmer of self-awareness. They are miserable with themselves, because they cannot be satisfied with anything on this earth. They don't yet realize that what they need is a living relationship with Jesus Christ. They blame all their misery on others around them — the job, the house, the in-laws, the children, or the neighbors. You may have some one in your life who is blaming you for his or her unhappiness, especially if you have become a Christian and they are still in "the world." I pray that you are enough aware of your Self and the TRUTH OF LIFE to know that we are each responsible for our own feelings and responses. There is no one who can make us either happy or unhappy. Nor are we able to make another person happy or unhappy. We either have the inner capacity for happiness or we do not. It does not come from the outside. It comes from within. Happiness and joy are responses of the soul. They have to be released from the innermost parts and are merely exhibited outwardly. They do not come from the outer influences.

This is such a tremendous truth and one which is so simple that it is often overlooked. Many people are burdened because they feel they are responsible to make someone happy . . . perhaps an unsaved loved one. That unsaved person is never going to find happiness while they are looking for it in the world. There are times when we must be what I call "divinely selfish" and step back in order to allow that loved one to suffer so that he or she will have the same opportunity to awaken to their need for Christ as we had. The awakened soul has something better than happiness . . . something not dependent upon the outer world or its fluctuating circumstances or upon the inconstancy of another

person. The awakened soul has joy unspeakable and full of
glory. But even this precious joy is only a prelude to the *bliss*
we will experience on that day when we see Him face to face.

The beginning of understanding comes when we quit
deluding ourselves to the reason of our suffering. We need to
admit to ourselves, first of all, that we are in pain and then
drink that bitter cup to the dregs. We must become fully
cognizant of all the heartache, all the depth of despair, and
all the physical limitations we must endure. *See all of it. Feel
all of it. Live all of it.* Go with it to the last degree. Let it
hurt as deeply as it can. And then reach into the farthest
pocket of pain hidden in the dark recesses of your soul
and yank it out.

You won't lose your mind. Some who have experienced
a mental breakdown, did so because they refused to feel their
pain. Some have chosen to retreat into a world of illusion and
dreams. Others have fractured into pieces rather than face the
reality of their painful experience. Still others have allowed
deep inner pain to transfer to their bodies rather than deal
with that mental anguish.

The most painful experience I ever had to go through was
losing my six-year old son who drowned in a well on my
parents' farm. When I saw his lifeless body lifted out of that
old cistern I ran screaming until I lost consciousness.

You mothers who are cuddling your children to your
breast right now can imagine what a terrible thing this would
be. Nothing could be worse. It was as if some vital organ in
the center of my being had been cut out and I was left with a
horrible bloody void which would never again be filled.

But I didn't try to avoid that pain. I was only twenty-seven years old, but, by the help of the Lord and His wisdom, I was guided step by step through that awful adjustment of loss, guilt, horror, confusion, self-doubt, self-pity, fear and the tangled mass of other thoughts and emotions which imprison a person who has suddenly lost a loved one due to a tragic accident. I never prayed for any of the pain to be removed from me.

Under the Lord's guidance, I knew that to push this experience into a forgotten corner of my soul would later on cause me either physical, mental or spiritual problems. I sensed even then, when all my future days were shrouded behind a gray cloud, that I had a higher calling and, therefore, I could not encumber my soul with grim, bitter memories of the past.

Instead, I prayed that God would give me the strength to be able to bear every microgram of pain that was in that experience so that I could learn enough from it that I would never have to go through anything like that again. I prayed that God would enlighten me through that season of grief so that the remainder of my life would be a memorial for the precious child I lost. The best way to do that was to *dedicate my life to Christ.*

Seven months after that tragic day, I was completely delivered from pain and grief and the hardest trial put before me became a time of decision for dedication. Paul said, *"For godly grief produces a repentance that leads to salvation and brings no regret, but worldly grief produces death."* (2 Cor. 7:10 R.S.V.)

It was through this tremendous scathing, that my soul was awakened. My religious disciplines were replaced with a personal experience with Jesus, my Lord and Savior. My point of focus was thereafter changed from this temporal world of death and decay to the spiritual world where life goes on eternally. I learned, beyond a shadow of a doubt, that there is no real death, neither for believers nor non-believers. I learned that the way we live here determines only the place where we shall live eternally when we have separated from this house of clay.

The Lord impressed upon me, at an early age, that the worst pain we can possibly suffer is that which comes from trying to avoid feeling pain. The horrible feeling of *dis-ease* within, which comes from trying to avoid confrontation with those stark realities of our revealed, carnal self, is the worst pain in the world. We can't find peace or happiness with anything or anyone. We go about with the awareness that some big bogeyman is about to jump out at us from behind the next bush.

Also, we can be extremely vulnerable during the times when we are being called into greater spiritual growth. Temptations will be thrown before us, by the enemy, to offer us an alternative to the pain which comes from facing ourselves. How often we have seen someone react to a tragedy by turning to some sin or vice. Satan was there offering an array of buffers from his kingdom.

Don't be afraid of hurting. When you discover and admit to yourself that you are suffering *dis-ease* in your spirit, take it before the Lord. Ask Him to teach you and strengthen you in this situation. When I see trouble coming, I don't panic and pray, "Oh, don't let it happen, Lord, don't let it happen!" But for a miracle of God, it's too late to pray that it won't happen. Remember, everything that happens to us today was set in motion in the past by ourselves. (See Matt. 7:26) Now is the time to pray for strength, wisdom and grace to be able to endure it!

Allow yourself to drink deep of the cup of sorrows while it is yours to drink. No matter how bitter the brew, drink it all. As your soul is retching from that most miserable concoction, pray God that the Holy Spirit brings to your awareness every tiny little act of spiritual rebellion of which you have been guilty, that which has helped shape this present situation.

As you confess and receive forgiveness from our Lord Jesus Christ, that bitter herb can be a catharsis which can cleanse your soul forever. Once all the contamination of the past is washed away, you need never again accumulate such debris. Each time you fall, go to the Lord immediately and ask for the cleansing which comes from being under His precious shed blood. Born-again believers have not only the privilege of doing this, but also, they have the responsibility to do it. We cannot be all that we were intended to be in Christ Jesus if we are suffering from guilt complexes. Even though we have forgiveness for all sins committed before our conversion, a great number of people have difficulty forgiving themselves for their rebellious acts prior to conversion.

When my marriage of eighteen years came to an end, I learned first-hand how the Holy Spirit works to free us from the bondage of unforgiveness.

I had believed before the separation that all the fault lay on the other side and I was just the poor innocent victim of an unChristian attack. I was ready and anxious for the marriage to end. I had suffered enough, I declared. But, I was totally unprepared for the suffering of loss which followed. It was the second most difficult time of my life. But I drank the whole cup, down to the dregs and the most amazing thing happened.

When I least expected it, there would be a replay in my mind of some incident which had taken place years before. I would view it with the dispassionate wisdom of the Lord. From His point of view, I saw things differently. I saw how many times I had had the opportunity of turning the direction of our lives and I either couldn't see it or refused to see it. But during the grieving period I saw it as the Lord must have viewed the situation. I saw that I was not the innocent victim after all. We each had a part to play and we played it . . . out of selfishness and bitterness, ignorantly and blindly and without real love. I hurt when I remembered all that I had contributed to the failure of our marriage. One by one the incidents of eighteen years floated up before my mind. It was truly my "Day of Judgement" and I was given opportunity to be the judge.

When all the 'prisoners' held in the dungeon of my subconscious mind were brought up before the judgement seat (my enlightened consciousness) I had the power to either confine these memories of my mistakes and failures within the depths of my soul, or release them. I chose to release them; to tear down the strongholds these erroneous thoughts had built, years before, through anger, hurt and rejection. I decided I didn't need to keep these memories alive within me any longer.

When we realize today that what we did yesterday was wrong, we begin to grow. When I realized my error the result was a broken spirit and a contrite heart. I knew, as I never could have known without this painful experience of failure, that *I* needed the mercy of God and the forgiveness through Christ Jesus. *I* needed His redemptive sacrifice on the cross. *I* needed the blood sacrifice which reinstated me to the Father hundreds of years before my moment of need. And when all of this glorious reality hit me, it shattered into billions of atoms which would be dispersed into the ethers forever all that I was before without Him. And it was only then, after all that, that the Lord was able to lift me up and make a new creation out of me, giving me a new heart and a new mind. All the former things were passed away. And then, miracle of miracles, the Holy Spirit entered into me to dwell in my heart!

Self-awareness begins with that moment of conversion when the Lord becomes real to us in a personal way *"to open their eyes, and to turn them from darkness to light and from the power of Satan unto God, that they may receive forgiveness of sins and inheritance among them which are sanctified by faith that is in me."* (Acts 26:18)

"To open their eyes," Jesus said. That would imply that, until the time of our conversion, we did not have our eyes opened. That perhaps we were sleep-walkers, moving about with neither awareness nor understanding of the trials which beset us.

Self-awareness can be developed by going over the events of the day before falling asleep at night. In the secrecy of our minds we can afford to be utterly honest as we view everything which happened to us that day. Was it a good day or fraught with confusion, disappointment and chaos? Honestly ask yourself what part you played in the confusion and how you might have turned it aside by responding differently. Candidly, we need to confront ourselves with this probing question time and again, "What did I do to bring this condition upon myself?" Bear in mind, the truth is that it could not have come into our life if we did not have the corresponding negativity to attract it.

Jesus said, " . . . *When thine eye is single, thy whole body also is full of light; but when thine eye is evil, thy body also is full of darkness."* (Luke 11:34)

Carl Jung, Swiss psychologist whose priceless contributions to his field of study have enriched our own understanding of the human psyche, spoke of the soul as consisting of two complimentary but antithetical spheres, the consciousness and the unconsciousness. Interestingly, he considered the realm of consciousness to be light and the realm of the unconscious to be darkness. He appointed to the psyche (or soul) four basic functions: thinking, feeling, sensation, and intuition. He further taught that if all these functions of the soul would be raised to consciousness, the whole sphere of the inner man would be raised to light and there would be no darkness in him. He would, at that point, according to

Jung's musing, cast off the last "earthly vestige" and thereby would be a complete being.

The Apostle Paul said, " . . . *be ye transformed by the renewing of your mind . . .* " (Rom. 12:2) The transforming work, therefore, is our responsibility. We must exercise our "will" to a higher level of consciousness, coming up out of the darkness of our lower nature into the light of the "spirit man." We should focus our will, with concentrated effort, upon whatsoever is true, positive, good report, edifying and virtuous. The primary change in consciousness will be followed, in due time, with a change in our behavior.

Again, we see that our manifested life reflects our level of consciousness. From the application of our will we shall experience life at whatever level we direct. That is why two people, living in the same house, eating at the same table, even sleeping in the same bed, may be living realms apart. One may live as in heaven while the other wrestles with the specters of hell. Each has ordered his or her life experience by what he determines with his level of consciousness. But the one hovering near the brink can be lifted up to sit in heavenly places when he focuses his will to a higher level of consciousness by sincerely accepting and declaring Jesus as his Lord and Savior.

We do not invoke the heavenly kingdom with a few well-worded decrees. We do no more than begin to prepare the mind to peel away layer upon layer of delusion which has so covered his original being that it is nearly misshapen beyond identification. But it is a place to begin. We recognize first and foremost the duality of our nature, claim that image made in the likeness of God (which is the absolute and true image) and gradually dispose and disclaim that which is not part of God's creation.

It would be a gross misrepresentation if I would say that applying one's self to the positive attributes of the higher consciousness would rescue us forever from the foreboding shadows of the unconscious which cause us to react in a compulsive-obsessive manner.

Training the intellect into a positive thought pattern is merely the discipline which prepares us for the Holy Work to begin. We must not believe that becoming baptized by the Holy Spirit preempts this inner work — to the contrary. I believe I have had more memories from my near-forgotten childhood since I have been baptized by the Spirit of God. I consider this to be healthy. Each time the Lord reveals to me the error of my ways, I am elated, because the more of the carnal self that is removed from me, the closer the Lord is. It is as if my real inner self has been hidden by enumerous veils. Each veil is a representation of some delusion, iniquity or ego crutch that I thought I had to have to survive. But each veil has separated me from the love of Christ. He has been outside all those veils and I could hear Him, but I couldn't see Him. Now as I am permitting the Holy Spirit to reveal the truth to me, the veils are being lifted and I can see the radiance of my Lord and I can dimly make out His appearance. He is altogether lovely! But I want to see more and more of Him and I want so much to come into the fullness of His radiance that I am not concerned about protecting my ego any longer.

I am willing for the purging; prepared for the cleansing of the Holy of Holies, and the tearing down of idols and the burning of the bones of dead priests. (See 2 Chron. 34)

We, Christians, are called to prepare ourselves to be a Church ablaze with Glory of the Lord. It is so thrilling to see the "numbers" which are being added to the "Body of Christ," daily, and the zeal which has been placed within them to do mighty works. We are on the verge of a spiritual explosion and we can feel the rumblings moving on the earth as the Power builds. There is such anticipation in the air of something tremendous about to take place. At times I don't want to go to sleep because I might miss something.

"If a man therefore purge himself from these, he shall be a vessel unto honor, sanctified, and meet for the master's use and prepared unto every good work." (2 Tim. 2:21) Those who are truly called according to His purpose are being led by the Spirit into a deeper, consecrated walk. The cleansing with hyssop is taking place. Not in order to precipitate a new car, or a house, or money or prestige. Not to accumulate material goods, or loving relationships, or admiration from the crowds. Nor to have a place of honor among men for our dedication and good works. No. Those who are permitting the purification to take place within them are doing so to be able to withstand the darkness up ahead. We are being strengthened now to endure the difficult times which are coming upon the earth. We are overcoming the flesh desires now while it is still day so that we will not be tempted when nighttime comes.

"Beloved, now are we the sons of God, and it doth not

*yet appear what we shall be: but we know that, when he shall
appear, we shall be like him; for we shall see him as he is.
And every man that hath this hope in him purifieth himself,
even as he is pure."* (1 John 3:2-3)

Therefore *". . . Cleanse your hands, ye sinners; and purify
your hearts, ye doubleminded."* (James 4:8) *". . . for as he
thinketh in his heart, so is he . . . "* (Prov. 23:7)

5

Did The Devil Make You Do It?

Cynthia K. is an honest, agreeable, soft-spoken woman, who, although crippled with rheumatoid arthritis in her retirement years, busies herself "doing good works." She visits the sick, makes surprise casseroles for a working mother, buys clothes at a thrift shop for the needy and waits hand and foot on those less able than herself. No matter how unpleasant a situation might be, she wears a perpetual expression of beatitude upon her face and manages to find something good to say about everyone.

Cynthia's choice of affliction tells a great deal about her. She was reared by strict, unaffectionate parents who enforced Puritannical values of good Christian living; "hard work, save money and don't be frivolous. And . . . learn to control your emotions!" Cynthia had followed those dictates without question even though she rebelled inwardly and resented having someone prescribe how she should live her life. All the emotions engendered by unjudicial and incompassionate RULES had to be pushed down again and again.

When she became of age, Cynthia moved away . . . far away. There she set up her own business. She became very successful, married, and had children. Most of her life she was the sole means of support for her family. But she didn't complain but kept her feelings locked up inside.

Although she worked many long hours each day she managed both business and home. Evenings were usually spent doing books of her business long after everyone else was in bed. It was not unusual for her to then close up her ledgers, don her apron and whip up a surprise batch of date bars to surprise her family when they got up in the morning.

Years passed, her children married and moved away, her husband died, and the responsibilities of business and competition with younger competitors was becoming too much for her. She became anxious and perhaps a little fearful, so when her daughter persuaded Cynthia to come live with her, the move to a distant state began the final phase of Cynthia's life.

It soon became evident that the son-in-law didn't want her there. He was domineering and unkind. He had strict rules which the women had to obey. He decided what they were to eat, when they would go to bed and even what they could read. Cynthia swallowed every protest. Within six months, she was afflicted with the painfully swollen joints of rheumatoid arthiritis.

All the anger she had swallowed as a child was rekindled under the domination of her son-in-law. But she wouldn't argue or defend her own rights. Nor would she disappoint her daughter by moving into an apartment of her own. She felt trapped in a situation totally unpleasant to herself but out of the lifelong habit of yielding to the wishes of someone else, she would make no effort to change the situation.

The unexpressed anger she felt toward her son-in-law for his assuming control over her life stirred the dying embers of the old feelings of inferiority and incompetency she had felt as a child. The situation and its resulting response caused her to loose all the successes she had known, all the challenges she met and overcame, all the independence of action and thought she had established — her self respect. She was reduced to reliving what she had known as a child and she resented it. The conflict of these powerful emotions raging inside her precipitated the crippling disease of arthritis.

Current studies in the field of adrenalectomy and the influence of stress indicates that negative emotions can precipitate illness while positive emotions can keep us healthy. Joan Arehart-Treichel in her recent book "BIOTYPES" * explains: "Positive emotions are known to lower adrenal steroid hormones while negative emotions are known to raise them and elevated adrenal steroid hormones are capable of depressing the immune system's ability to fight disease. What's more, a feeling of helplessness . . . has been shown to impair the body's immune system, whereas the opposite emotion — belief that one can cope — does not have this effect. Depression and grief, two other well-documented predisposers to disease, have also been shown to depress the immune system."

Mrs. Arehart-Treichel goes on to explain that repressed emotions appear to prepare people for disease more fre-

* Biotypes by Joan Arehart-Treichel
  Reprinted by permission of Time Books, a division of Quadrangle/The New York Times Book Co., Inc.

quently than those negative emotions which we express openly. Evidence of this shows up palpably when tests indicate a high level of an antibody called IgA when a person suppresses anger. It may be that this antibody alteration is responsible for lowering the immune system of an angry individual which then results in an illness.

Many of our emotions are expressed physically and we don't give it a second thought. We turn red when we are angry, white with fear, our eyes fill with tears at the thought of something sad, ears turn red with embarrassment, we break out in a sweat with nervousness, we get hot, or cold, we tremble, shake, get weak in the knees and sometimes break out in a rash . . . all because of what we are experiencing emotionally! These observations are part of our everyday experience. Is it inconceivable, therefore, to speculate that some of our more serious ailments have been produced by our emotions at the unconscious level?

Freud introduced the concept that when bodily symptoms develop in response to *chronic* emotional conflicts we have what is termed conversion hysteria. One of the most important discoveries Sigmund Freud made was that when emotion is not expressed and relieved through normal means, voluntarily, it can become the source of chronic mental or physical disorder.

We have emotions which we determine to be inappropriate to the image we wish to project. We refuse to allow these emotions to be expressed in our normal interactions with others in order to maintain the status quo of the relationship. But the unexpressed emotions have produced a tremendous energy which must somehow be expended. If expression of this energy is cut off from the consciousness, where it cannot be worked off through physical activity, tensions in the body develop which have an adverse reaction on every muscle and nerve ending and every internal organ.

Pauline G. married a man of whom her parents vehemently disapproved. Not long after the nuptials, all the dire predictions of her parents toward her husband proved to be true. He had a violent temper, insatiable lust and pathological tendencies in more than one area. But Pauline continued in the marriage, hiding from everyone the truth of what her marriage was like.

Fear for her life mounted as her husband's pathology increased. One night, in a burst of violent anger, he threatened her with a gun, placing it against her head while she was sleeping. She awakened, somehow freed herself from him and fled the house. She was found in the morning, incoherently babbling undecipherable sounds. Even then, after all she had been through for 15 years, she could not tell anyone . . . at least not in a language they could understand.

We can see by these two examples that some good, conscientious people can suffer more serious complaints than those who just don't care. "Good" people frequently find themselves in situations where they are trying to serve the demands of someone else while at the same time suppressing the desire to do what they instinctively know is best for them.

It is this conflict (and the denial of it) which causes much of the physical distress good people suffer. It is doing what we don't want to do and inwardly resenting it. It is telling ourselves to turn the other cheek when what we want to do is "bop the other fellow in the nose."

A recent retrospective study found that at least 65% of those diagnosed as "anxious" complained of aching muscles and physical tension rather than an emotional conflict. This confirmed earlier reports that a high level of emotional tension is reflected in a heightened muscular tension.

Oftentimes, the placement of these musculoskeletal symptoms gives some clue as to the inner problem which the patient is not able to identify. A stiff neck, for instance, might be a clue that the patient doesn't want to face the problem which is causing the emotional conflict. Excruciating leg cramps in one woman served to underline her statement, "I can't stand it anymore" in reference to her husband's drinking problem. Another woman developed such a painful affliction in her shoulders soon after her husband's death that she wasn't able to raise her arms to comb her hair or dress herself. This indicated her deep fear of having to "shoulder responsibility" now that she was alone.

A man, having married right out of high school and having six children before he was twenty-five, worked hard and long hours for many years; getting all the children through the lower grades of school and providing not only necessities but many more luxuries than most kids expect or warrant. He had one dream which kept him going . . . that of retiring from the mill at an early age and getting a little farm in the country where he would be able to work at his own pace doing the things he enjoyed most. But the wife and children had other ideas. College was a must for all of them. He soon became chronically incapacitated for months at a time with such excruciating back pain. He could barely walk from bed to bathroom, yet physical examinations showed no physical explanation for his problem. An extensive interview with the doctor revealed he had a deeply hidden resentment of having "to carry all these people on my back."

Dr. Dunbar, in her book "MIND AND BODY: PSYCHOMATIC MEDICINE" says: "The chooser of symptoms does not set out with malice aforethought. There must be a real emotional need for illness first. Then on the borderline between the known and the forgotten the choice of symptom will be made."

"Before it does permanent damage to the body, the emotional need for the illness must be removed. It can be done only if the victim first understands just what has roused the need and faces up to the situation. Self-understanding is not always the most pleasant thing in the world for anyone. But it may be worth the price. It may help remove the cause along with the symptoms."

In Dr. Dunbar's perceptive observation lies the key to why people do not always get their healing in the prayer line despite the faith, the annointing, the word and the prayers!

Paul said, *"When I was a child, I spake as a child, I understood as a child, I thought as a child: but when I became a man, I put away childish things."* (1 Cor. 13:11) The notion that we are sick because Satan has made us sick is a childish thing which those who are becoming mature in the Word should be ready to put away.

It is true enough that people are perishing for lack of

knowledge and many are the born-again believers who have
not fed long enough upon the Word to know what the truth
is. And what is the teaching which leads believers away from
the work of overcoming their carnal natures? *It is the belief
that all our afflictions and distresses are put upon us by
Satan.*

This factious belief keeps the children of God from accepting the responsibility of the circumstances in their lives which
they have precipitated by living out of harmony with Him.
And much of this disharmony isn't outright sin or open
rebellion. Sometimes the disharmony is a current of unrest
deep within the soul because we are sacrificing ourselves to
do what others expect us to do. But if we can be made to
believe that we are mere ropes in a tug-of-war between the
forces of good and evil and that we are totally innocent of
any consequences, either good or bad, we can be kept from
learning the truth of our nature and assuming the power
we have been given by Christ Jesus.

As long as Christians are bound by the belief that they are
helpless pawns in the hands of intangible, invisible forces far
beyond their control, they will never grow in power nor start
DEMONSTRATING victory in Christ. What is more, the very
feeling of helplessness in the face of overwhelming power
can precipitate deadly disease.

Jesus *has* overcome powers and principalities and princes
of darkness. He holds the keys. He has bequeathed that power
and authority to us as believers. Satan can lie to us and tell us
differently, but since we all know he is a liar and the father
of lies, why is anyone listening to him? I am delivered! So are

you . . . if you want to be!

There is only One God, One Creator, One who has omnipotent power and that is Jehovah God. Jesus said, *"All power
is given unto me in heaven and in earth."* (Matt. 28:18) Is
Jesus a liar? Of course not ! Then why do Christians assign
power unto Satan when Jesus took it ALL away?

Satan has no power to either create or destroy in the life
of the born-again believer. Instead of going around declaring
that Satan did this or that to us, we should be *"Giving thanks
unto the Father, which hath made us meet to be partakers
of the inheritance of the saints in light. Who hath delivered
us from the power of darkness, and hath translated us into
the kingdom of his dear Son: . . . "* (Col. 1:12-13)

If Satan has power over us it is because we give him the
power by opening our minds to negativity and fear. We begin
to think we are powerless in the face of circumstances and
so we are. We forget that we are children of Light which
Satan and his cohorts are unable to approach. Therefore, the
Satanic influence people find in their lives may be an influence stemming from the psychologically damaged lower self
which precipitates its own failures, rejections, calamities
and afflictions.

That Satan is a real influence and spirit being is not to be
argued, for even the most astute scholars concede their belief
in such; but every day, in a thousand ways, we give ourselves
to him.

The Biblical representation of Satan is: the tempter, the
prince of demons, source of demonical possession, god of the
underworld, prince of the power of the air, disguised as an

angel of light, an adversary, the deceiver of the whole world,
the great dragon, the old serpent, the seducer of Adam and
Eve, Paul's thorn in the flesh, the moving spirit of apostasy,
a roaring lion, wiley, the spirit that works in the disobedient,
one who takes advantage of Christians. He was able to: put
betrayal into the heart of Judas, pervert the Scriptures,
hinder Paul's missionary plans, cause Ananias to lie, produce
false miracles, move David to sin, cause Job's troubles, be an
adversary to Joshua and be called the father of evil men.

BUT . . . he will flee, if resisted, and is overcome by faith.
Jesus triumphed over him, and broke the bonds he had upon
the world. And, since Jesus has lifted the born-again believer
up with Him to high heavenly places where Satan has no
power over us, he cannot touch us!

But we can invite him in. We do that by the thoughts we
entertain. Satan attacks us through our minds. If he cannot
get a foothold in our minds, he cannot influence us at all. So
once again, the responsibility falls back on us. If we claim
that Satan has attacked us, or afflicted us or led us into
temptation, we are admitting that we took our eyes off Jesus
and started entertaining thoughts which were out of harmony
with the nature of God.

But most people do not keep watch over their thoughts
or the workings of their minds so that everything is kept in
subjection to Christ. We allow ourselves to foster hurts, to
dwell over circumstances which are ancient history, to blow
things up out of proportion and make much out of little, to
be suspicious of the intentions of others, to carry forth a bad
report, to look for evil rather than good, and to talk about,

and to read about and listen to reports on the evil of the children of darkness.

When we turn our thoughts toward the carnal life and away from Jesus Christ, Satan is prepared to rush in, add to our already-existing negativity with his lies and enticements and begin working his deceit to our total disadvantage.

Satan does not make us sick. He tempts us, deceives us, accuses us by broadcasting thoughts of worry, anger, resentment, anxiety, fear, and self-pity into our minds until we permit our emotions and thoughts to manifest afflictions which we subconsciously feel the need to suffer. As a spirit-being, Satan is limited to working in the non-physical world so he didn't push you off the porch or make your car break down or cause the sewer to back up. Every time you make a claim such as that, you are honoring the devil. You are speaking his name and giving him the negative glory for the circumstances in your life when what you should be sending forth as a righteous decree is: THERE IS BUT ONE POWER IN MY LIFE, AND THAT IS ALMIGHTY GOD, AS REVEALED TO ME THROUGH JESUS CHRIST. HIM ONLY DO I SERVE.

If we become suddenly ill and think it is a Satanic attack, all we have to do is rebuke him in the name of Jesus and the symptoms will disappear immediately. If they don't, then we must look to ourselves for the cause of the affliction which will, if we are seeking God's wisdom, correct us and purge us of unrighteousness.

We can't become the fullness of Christ until we have emptied out all the garbage we have collected in the inner self.

And it is impossible to express true love for our fellowman
— or even our mates — when we are subconsciously bound
by our own forgotten failures, rejections, sins and prejudices.
Where our hearts are crammed full of congealed feelings of
insufficiencies which we are trying to hide from the world,
there is no room left for the Word to dwell in us richly. There
is no way that we can indefinitely hide what we really are
inside, " . . . *for out of the abundance of the heart, the
mouth speaketh.*" (Matt. 12:34) When we least expect it,
the old man will show himself alive and still fighting for expression. Then the word we speak will return unto Him
void because our emotion will nullify it.

That is why it is so important to get the whole act together;
head and heart in submission only unto Him. He will make of
us a vessel unto honor *if* we are willing to allow it to be. But
there are things in us which we must be willing to sacrifice:
all our crutches and excuses and alibis and intellectual explanations. Then we shall start getting results from prayer.

As Dr. Dunbar said, the emotional need for the illness
must be removed before the body can be healed. An interesting case is that of a young woman who is frequently
in the hospital — being tested for some strange, elusive
malady. She has real, physical symptoms which, for years,
doctors have been unable to group under one nomenclature.
So serious are some of her complaints, that, if her ailment
had not been psychogenic in nature, she would have been
dead years ago. Yet she continues on, amazingly healthy for
as sick as she is. She had been given up for adoption at birth,
never saw her real mother, was placed in a series of foster

homes until she was adopted at the age of ten. From that time on, she had a good, secure life with a wonderful family. But what anxieties, fear, insecurities, sense of abandonment, grief and aloneness marked that infant at birth which was transmitted to her flesh some thirty years later?

Two San Francisco cardiologists, who undertook a study to determine the cause of heart attacks, discovered that personality had more to do with fatal disease than obesity, cigarette smoking, lack of exercise or stress. Their study further indicated that people who are deeply "religious" have a rare incidence of heart attacks. It seems that those who are more interested in the life hereafter adapt themselves better to stress.

In Hebrew the word "devil" is translated "ayin" which means: eye, or foundation, signifying the external or superficial appearance of things and the transiency of the finite world. Things are not as they appear to us through the deceiver of the eye. The eye tells us that each of us is flesh and blood, that what we see is real, and in order to continue living, we must have these physical bodies. If we believe what the eye tells us, we will live to the flesh. Since spiritual things cannot be seen, they are not real to the one who believes only what his eye tells him. Even though our space equipment has rended the skies, heaven has remained undiscovered. The spirit and soul of man defies observation. Is this to say that neither heaven nor the spirit of man exists? Of course not. Yet wouldn't the "deceiver" have you believe just that? If there was no heaven, there would be no need of sanctification and holiness in the flesh.

Further definition of the Hebrew word for "devil" implies that it personifies the false conception that man is bound by material conditions, that he is a slave to circumstances and a sport of fate. "Devil" is also defined as sensation. If, through lack of knowledge, we don't understand the sensation we are feeling, it can lead us into sin. An example would be the sensation of hunger even though a person has eaten adequately. Without understanding, he feeds the sensation of hunger until he is guilty of gluttony, when in fact, the sensation he feels might be hunger for a meaningful relationship with another person.

Every single device of the devil can be turned around and used for our further growth in the spirit. We can grow to tremendous spiritual height in the wake of adversity, we can use failure as a stepping stone to greater success, and when we are about to be crushed by the weight of lies and delusion we can more easily awaken to the strength and power of our Lord to do battle on our behalf. Then, we experience renewal instead of defeat.

Most of us make no real effort to be free of the enemy's influence until we feel we have run out of ability to strive. We actually have to be "sick unto death" sometimes, before we fight to become well. And most of us will continue in the chains of Satan, interminably, unless we feel the shackles rubbing us raw. Then, and only then, do people determine to break free. And, when we make that determination, we find, to our great amazement, the chains have been so loose we could have escaped them at any time. We were only imprisoned because we believed ourselves to be.

Satan is evident in his work as the deceiving phase of our minds. This can take various forms. Ideas we hold dear which are in opposition to the Word of God is really the devil at work. He works in us as egotism, a puffed-up personality, self-depreciation, self-pity, a desire to control others, avoiding responsibility, slothfulness, a negative outlook on life and a strong attachment to sense consciousness.

Satan also works in the minds of men by making them believe that they are so evil there is no hope for them or that they are so smart they don't need a Sovereign God. Satan has taken control of a person when he rebels against God when he is confronted with hard experiences. And the one who believes there is no God is, of course, under the deceptive influence of Satan.

"And the seventy returned again with joy, saying, Lord, even the devils are subject unto us through thy name. And he said unto them, I beheld Satan as lightning fallen from heaven." (Luke 10:17-18)

Heaven is a place of perfect harmony. When our thoughts are in submission to God, our minds can be in heavenly places. But when we permit thoughts which are out of alignment with the nature of God, we have permitted Satan to enter into our minds and there is the "war in heaven." When this occurs, we have the authority to use the name of Jesus Christ and Satan must depart from influencing our thought processes. He has fallen from "heaven" as lightning.

Lightning is produced and discharged without warning. It is a tremendous force but it is unharnessed, so its potential is wasted. Lightning released in heaven (from cloud to cloud) is harmless, but when lightning strikes the earth, it can kill, maim, and destroy.

Satan can project his thoughts into our minds. He will probably never stop trying. And if you wear the helmet of faith all day to keep him away from your mind, you'll find he will try to sneak in when you are sleeping. But the blood of Jesus will keep our minds covered so that we will know his influence and take authority over it. He is then powerless to do anything to a blood-bought child of God.

But if you permit him to plant thoughts in your mind which are in conflict with God's mind, those thoughts can strike like lightning into your flesh, causing you to become afflicted. If you speak the Name of Jesus at the very onset of a Satanic idea, Satan must "fall."

It is interesting to note, also, that in the many sources researched to find the nuances of the meaning of Satan and devil, the Greek word that is translated in Luke 4:1-13 means accuser or the "critical one." We have one word in the English language which comes closest to the Greek word and that is *personality*.

Personality is defined as the sum of characteristics which constitutes an individual. Personality is not part of the permanent being created in the image of God. Personality is temporal and transient, relating only to this phase of earth life. And this personality can be a "devil" to the more permanent part of ourselves — our souls. The personality can be strong enough to completely dominate the physical vehicle, allowing the spirit man little or no expression. Yet, even in this behavior we see a contra-indication, because it is usually in the under-developed ego that this behavior appears.

Those who have permitted the healthy development of the personality at the intellectual, social and spiritual levels are individualistic people who are not threatened by ego-sacrificing which is necessary to develop spiritually. They are not governed by the negative mores or influences of the masses. They respond to a higher calling and dare to answer that call — even if it means being alone.

Carl Jung, in "DEVELOPMENT OF PERSONALITY" explains, "What is it, in the end, that induces a man to go his own way and to rise out of unconscious identity with the mass as out of a swathing mist? Not necessity, for necessity comes to many and they all take refuge in convention. Not moral decision, for nine times out of ten we decide for convention, likewise. What is it then, that inexorably tips the scales in favour of the extraordinary?

It is what is commonly called *vocation*: an irrational factor that destines a man to emancipate himself from the herd and from its well-worn paths. True personality is always a vocation and puts its trust in it as in God, despite its being, as the ordinary man would say, only a personal feeling. But vocation acts like a law of God from which there is no escape. The fact that many a man who goes his own way ends in ruin means nothing to one who has a vocation. He *must* obey his own law. Anyone with a vocation hears the voice of the inner man: He is *called!*"

Jung explains that the original meaning of "to have a vocation" is "to be addressed by a voice." Those who have heard the voice of the inner man understand full well there-

fore the meaning of having a vocation while those who have
it not cannot understand however frequently it is explained.

"The smaller the personality, the dimmer and more
unconscious it (the voice of the inner man) becomes, until
finally it merges indistinguishably with the surrounding
society, thus surrendering its own wholeness and dissolving
into the wholeness of the group. In the place of the inner
voice there is the voice of the group with its conventions,
and vocation is replaced by collective necessities. But even
in this unconscious social condition there are not a few who
are called awake by the summons of the voice, whereupon
they are at once set apart from the others, feeling themselves
confronted with a problem about which the others know
nothing (from *Collected Works of C. G. Jung,* Volume 17,
Pantheon Books).

The work of Satan since the dawn of creation has been,
simply, ego-entrapment, and because we have been held
captive in such a tangled web, it has seemed impossible to
extricate ourselves so that we would be able to discover
". . . the hidden man of the heart, . . . " (1 Pet. 3:4)

We have all been in situations which have left negative
marks engraved upon the heart. These experiences have injured the immature ego of our childhood and left us with
feelings of inferiority, incompetence, unimportance, rejection and insecurity. Since we were "no good to begin with"
we later added sin.

In order for that struggling ego to survive these inner
wounds, defense mechanisms . . . designed for survival . . .
were put into operation. If we were made to feel inferior

by our circumstances, we adopted behavior which made us feel superior, or at least convinced others that we thought we were.

The obsessive-compulsive behavior patterns control the fragmented individual whose weakened ego is struggling to stay alive. They also serve to keep us defensively separated from our fellow man. Then we begin a process of behavior which keeps us from having that which we need most in order to become whole.

There are also side effects to this behavior pattern. We generally become angry, more at ourselves than anyone else, that we are permitting ourselves to be caught in this vortex. The anger produces guilt which makes us feel uneasy . . . with others, with ourselves and with God . . . and the uneasiness produces insecurity which then must be satisfied by the constant reassurances of those about us. When they are not, fear floods the inner consciousness, and that produces depression. And depression will result, sooner or later if allowed to persist, in physical or mental breakdown.

Depression is entering mentally into the vestibule of hell. It is standing in the dark and gloomy jaws of the inferno where you can meet no one but the cohorts of Satan. Most people enter into this gloomy passageway of their own free will because they are trying to get attention, trying to test someone's love and concern for them. It is a dangerous game to play. If you play it long enough, one of Satan's cohorts may notice you and coax you further into his kingdom. So, whatever your personality problem, whatever obsessive-compulsive behavior controls your life, fight for all you are worth against allowing yourself to become depressed.

No matter how dim the picture may seem, there is hope out of all the morass of mental tangle we have allowed to be created within us. One writer explains the bodily condition this way: "The body is not so fragile as we sometimes fear. It is capable of forceful resistance. It can be pushed far, very far, and still find resources to recover unless the spirit is broken or the body tissues are worn out . . . true recovery is . . . in our hands if we have the will."

And isn't that what healing is all about? An exercising of our *will* to live in health. Sometimes we think it is not God's will for us to be well when, in fact, it is not our will. We haven't become courageous enough to allow the cleansing within to take place. We may not like what we are but what we are is all we've got, we think, and maybe we'd better hang onto that flesh.

There have been a significant number of scientific studies and clinical observations, in recent years, to indicate that while there is a commonality of these different psychological profiles indicating a deep sense of worthlessness as the predisposer in most cases of psychosomatic illnesses, the patient can break that pattern of destructive behavior. We can't change the events of early life which caused us to feel worthless or insecure, but we can look them over objectively and see them in a new light and with new understanding, thereby discharging the emotional content of those early experiences.

The Book of Revelations is full of wonderful promises "to him that overcometh." Granted, the world abounds in temptations which we pray for power to overcome, but the greatest battle of overcoming takes place within ourselves.

It is frightening to begin releasing negative emotions which we have been bottling up all our lives. Our prime fear is that we will lose the love of those who are important to us if they know how ugly we feel inside. But the alternatives to this exposure as being less than perfect is to suffer the consequences of unexpressed anger and its resulting guilt.

An article entitled "FAITH HEALING" in the December 1973 issue of *The Journal of Nervous and Mental Disease* states that a number of born-again patients had experienced physical healing after their religious experience. These healings were not only of the less severe chronic complaints such as backache, ulcers, and asthma, but also of life-threatening diseases such as cancer and tuberculosis.

Being born-again of the Spirit of God . . . a true conversion of the inner man as well as the personality . . . receiving the new heart and new mind in Christ Jesus . . . is the best defense we have against the diseases of this world and the influence of Satan. *"We know that whosoever is born of God sinneth not; but he that is begotten of God keepeth himself, and that wicked one toucheth him not."* (1 John 5:18)

"Know thyself" was the admonition carved over the arch to the temple of the ancient Greek oracle. Though we respond to a Higher Calling than that of a forgotten mystic, the advise can be well taken, for it appears that we cannot be all that God intends us to be until we know ourselves. And as we permit the release of the debris of the unconscious mind under the cleansing, purging fire of the Holy Spirit, we shall then be able to be sanctified wholly and our whole *"spirit, soul, and body will be preserved blameless unto the coming of the Lord Jesus Christ."* (1 Thess. 5:23 Paraphrased)

6

I Will Declare The Decree.

As the wife of a successful businessman, it appeared that Irene S. had everything: beautiful home, expensive furniture, big car, designer clothes. However, there was a haunting look of sadness in her eyes which only hinted at the amount of suffering and disappointment she had known over the years.

She and her husband befriended me while I was still in high school, inviting me for dinners after church or taking me to special church functions. Not having any children of their own, they both were delighted when in the company of young people.

Irene confided to me the reason for her perpetual sadness. She had had several children, each of whom died within the first few years of his or her life. Irene had had even more pregnancies which terminated before the child was born. It had been exceptionally difficult for her, hungering for a child as she had been. Due to a severe heart condition, her doctor advised against any future pregnancies. Thus began a search for an adoptable child.

The search, however, became long and hard. Due to Irene's ill health, they were turned down by every legal adoption agency. But she didn't give up. Compromising her beliefs, she finally talked her husband into going through illegal channels.

Soon, a pink-wrapped bundle was being carried to church. Now that she had a precious baby girl, Irene never looked happier *or* healthier.

Then, four short years later, the baby's mother, now married and wanting the child she gave away, went to court to get custody of her child. The judge decided in favor of the natural mother, principally because of Irene's heart condition and the advancing years of her husband. Irene replied, "I can't swallow that."

Irene's minister was with her at the courthouse. He tried to counsel her, but she simply replied, "I can't swallow that!"

She said those words over and over again, and in the weeks which followed, she slipped deeper and deeper into depression. To everyone she met she related her heartbreaking story and her opinion of "the judge's bias against her."

Weeks later she went to church. During the service she wandered down the empty halls. When I saw her I thought I was seeing a spectre from the grave! She was so grotesquely thin and bore no resemblance to a human being! Her skin was gray and shrivelled. Her eyes so deeply sunken that she looked like a walking skeleton. Black circles framed her lifeless eyes. Many of her teeth had fallen out of their sockets. The hideous sight reminded me of those who had come out of concentration camps following World War II. "Irene! What happened to you?" I gasped. She whispered that she couldn't swallow.

For some strange reason her throat seemed to close up whenever she tried to eat. She couldn't swallow anything. At that time no one had heard of "anorexia nervosa," and she obviously had no thought of getting psychological help for her problem. She was "starving to death" right before our eyes. No one could do anything to help her. She had *spoken into existence* a condition which was destroying her. She finally died.

Without realizing what they are doing, people are quick to speak situations into existence. "He makes me sick!" "That burns me up!" "She turns my stomach!" "My boss makes my blood boil!" "That eats my heart out!" "I am going to blow my top!" "That drives me crazy!" "Everything gets on my nerves!" "I could commit murder!" "I can't stand this any longer!"

Every day, statements like these are peppered through conversations, with little understanding of what the speaker is calling forth for himself. Diabetes, high blood pressure, gastrointestinal problems, strokes, insanity, nervous conditions, ulcers and more.

"Woe unto them that decree unrighteous decrees, and that write grievousness which they have prescribed; . . . " (Isa. 10:1) Whether for good or ill, our words have power. We can actually speak into existence certain conditions in our lives. "The power of life and death is in the tongue." *"For by thy words thou shalt be justified, and by thy words thou shalt be condemned."* (Matt. 12:37)

God spoke the cosmos into being. With the Word, God made this universe as well as this planet we call "home." He spoke the rivers, seas, dry plains and rocky mountains into existence. He uttered a sound and there was light separating the darkness. And . . . our Lord Jesus Christ is "The Word"!

The power of God is hidden in the Word. Jesus, Who was God's power in the flesh, came to earth that we might partake of that power. We are made in His image. In the flesh we are an image misshapen as we are seen through the density of earth's carnal atmosphere. But, we discover we can be like Him. God is love, so we can be loving. God is mercy. We can be merciful. God is wisdom. We can be wise. God is forgiveness and we can be forgiving.

As pale mirror images of the Father who created us, we have power to speak things into existence. *"A good man out of the good treasure of the heart bringeth forth good things: and an evil man out of the evil treasure bringeth forth evil things . . . for out of the abundance of the heart, his mouth speaketh."* (Matt. 12:34-35)

Susan G. was always saying, "That drives me out of my mind!" Or, "Those people are going to drive me crazy!" She had a nervous breakdown when she was in her mid-fifties. Thirty years later, she is still decreeing insanity for herself. How sad!

I knew of several men who were always "blowing their tops" when things didn't go their way. Nearly every one of them has had a stroke, and two of them died in their forties!

Another dear woman, whose son had disappointed her, confessed to everyone that he had broken her heart. She died at the age of fifty-two with a massive coronary.

Although these anecdotes might sound like exaggerations, I assure you, they are not. *"That ye put off concerning the former conversation the old man, which is corrupt according to the deceitful lusts. Wherefore putting away lying, speak every man truth with his neighbor: for we are members one of another. Let no corrupt communication proceed out of your mouth, but that which is good to the use of edifying, that it may minister grace unto the hearers."* (Eph. 4:22, 25, 29).

Most of us realize that boasting will make one unpopular and such habits as carrying tales, gossiping, lying, criticizing, judging, and revealing secrets are obvious social misbehavior. But how many of us realize what action we set in motion when we decree an unrighteous decree? Are we aware that when we give voice to fear, evil, or negativity, we begin drawing these experiences to ourselves in the same manner that a magnet draws metal filings? Job warned, *"Thou shalt also decree a thing, and it shall be established unto thee: . . . "* (Job 22:28a) When we fear something we bring it upon ourselves.

How can this be? How can we . . . just by saying something or thinking something . . . bring a situation into existence? The Lord warned us that by the words of our mouths we shall be condemned and that we shall be held accountable for every idle word.

Our words condemn us because others can see what we've called forth into our own lives. We are made accountable for our words by having to live in the midst of what we have created.

Our Heavenly Father isn't being arbitrary. He established the laws which govern our universe. They are impersonal laws which apply to saint and sinner alike. When we speak, we are calling into effect these immutable laws of creation and, once set into motion, there is no stopping what we are calling forth. We made it and we have to live with it.

Just think, you form an idea in your mind, then you polarize that idea with your fervent desire. In due time the manifestation takes place. Thought alone can't bring forth creation. Neither can feeling alone create. It takes the unified activation of both.

Thought is considered a masculine activity while *feeling* or emotion is feminine. It takes male and female acting in unity to bring forth offspring and it takes thought and feeling for us to speak our creations into existence.

Everthing that was, is or ever shall be, exists right now in the ethers surrounding us. There is nothing new on earth or under heaven. God has made the basic ingredients for all things.

When you desire to create something, you form the idea of what you want, and through the activation of your thought processes, you generate the energy to draw to your thoughts the necessary atoms to build your creation. Remember, space is not a void, but the energy is latent until it is activated by an outside force. Your thoughts act as that motivating force. Your emotion regarding that thought germinates the energy.

You speak the word of creation, "Let there be . . . " and

the energy behind your idea merges with the power of your word, sending it out into this sea of cosmic energy. It travels rapidly, gathering speed as it travels, and since *like attracts like,* according to the law of magnetism, your idea and word collects and gathers similar words. This creative mass of atoms gains momentum as it travels at greater and greater speeds through space, producing more energy.

Interestingly, your creative words merge with the thoughts and words, sometimes careless words, of other individuals. This is in accordance with the *magnetic law of attraction.* When all the atoms which have been activated by similar thinking and feeling people cohese, a gigantic creation is formed. And, since everything eventually returns to its source of origin, our thoughts and words come back to us, increased a hundredfold. We and our co-creators have to live with what we have made. *"Cast thy bread upon the waters; for thou shalt find it after many days."* (Ecc. 11:1)

Our good comes back to us in the same manner. Everyone gets exactly what he has decreed by thought, word and deed. Everyone is in the place where he is supposed to be according to his level of consciousness and no one can have anything for which he has not developed the consciousness.

In other words, *we can't have health if our consciousness is geared for sickness.* We cannot be rich if we have consciousness only for lack and need. No one can take something away from another person and expect to keep what he has taken. If he had had consciousness for that particular thing it would have manifested itself in his own life. He wouldn't have had to take it from someone else.

Once we recognize this fundamental truth of the *Universal God,* Who has established the laws which govern all the limitless cosmos, we can finally begin the work of allowing His will to be on earth as it is in heaven. That world will be one of such harmony with the mind of God that there can be no sickness, tears, poverty or death. But first, our righteousness must exceed that of the Pharisees.

The Pharisees represent that part of our intellect which holds to the outward form of worship rather than entering into the spirit of worship. Our Pharasaical thoughts are the hardest to be overcome because they usually are spiritualized. Therefore, they have more power in and over us; that is, until we have that *inner witness* of the Holy Spirit. The ideas which spring forth from above are precious to us. We may guard them, superstitiously, even as the Pharisees guarded the numerous Levitical laws. The Pharisees resented He Who appeared ready to abolish the outer adherence to the law and spoke about the deeper meaning of the law. In the same manner, our intellectual minds rebel when we realize that all we need is fulfilled in Christ without the price required by the doctrinal practice of denominationalism. No wonder Jesus warned His disciples that in the latter days there would rise up many who had a form of religion but would deny the power behind it.

The only time I have been hospitalized was to give birth to my children and also after a near-fatal automobile accident. In retrospect, however, the collision . . . while appearing to be an accident . . . was in direct accordance with the Law of God.

My mother had been in an accident when she was nineteen years old and dating my dad. She had been thrown through the roof of my dad's brand new Model "A" Ford when the car skidded on a wet pavement on a bridge and then went over the side. Mother was in a coma for days. When she regained consciousness, it was discovered she was blind in one eye from a blood clot on the optic nerve. The blood clot later dissolved, but, needless to say, after such a traumatic experience, my mother was not a very relaxed traveller.

All my young life I had been taught, by my mother's reactions, that going for a ride in an automobile was just about the most terrifying thing a person could do. Going over bridges was like a horror unto death. If my dad drove faster than thirty miles an hour, my mother went into hysterics.

She'd scream and cry and stiffen up and brace herself. My three little sisters and I would sit on the back seat very still and wide-eyed and learn how to behave when we went for a Sunday afternoon drive.

Having learned my lesson well, I grew up terrified of cars and especially bridges. I never wanted to go anywhere, unless I could walk. One autumn we planned a little week-end trip, with the children, to visit some friends who lived about 200 miles away. The night before, as I was setting my hair, the enemy put the thought in my mind, "This is the last time you will have to set your hair!"

I froze in terror and pleaded to stay home. But I was talked out of my unfounded fear and we went. Coming back on Sunday afternoon, we were hit head-on in a five-car

collision and our Chevrolet was folded like an unused ac-
cordian. We had severe injuries but nothing compared to
what could have been if, through my fear, I had not been
praying constantly for the Lord to keep His hand over us.

The state trooper who investigated the accident broke
down and cried as he questioned me because, he said, it was
such a miracle that any of us got out of that mangled heap of
metal alive!

No one was killed! Neither the boy who caused the accident, nor the elderly man and woman he hit in the rear, who
were thrown out of control across the divided highway, nor
the people in front of us who were hit broadside, nor any
of the five of us who were hit head-on, nor the man and
woman who ran into the back of us when everything came
to such a screeching halt. It really was a miracle!

The first realization I had when I regained consciousness,
in the hospital, was that if God had wanted to take me in an
auto accident, He certainly had had His chance and since I
had survived, this apparently was not the way I was going to
depart from this world. I knew so little about God's promise
at that time. I really did not understand what was His will for
me. The ritualistic church I'd attended all my life didn't
equip a Christian to deal with life.

After this accident I realized that I need not fear traveling
in a car. But I learned something even more important. After
I was taken out of intensive care and put in a semi-private
room, I had a roommate, probably in her early 50's, who was
one of the most bitter-mouthed persons I had ever met. She
was awaiting surgery, but I suspected that her illness was not

the cause of her meanness. Her family members each had a stooped, dejected appearance worn by those who are under the scrutiny of a tyrant.

It was apparent she considered me an intruder into her domain. But, since my conversation was limited to nods and shrugs due to a badly chewed-up tongue, I was in no condition to force my company upon her. I listened to everything that went on on her side of the room. After all, what else did I have to do?

In time, I was able to piece together her story: The woman had her father living with her for many years, and was very devoted to him. Even though she had a family of her own, she never outgrew being "daddy's little girl." It was obvious that he had first place in her life. Then he got sick. It turned out to be cancer of the colon and she, dedicatedly, took care of him until the time of his death. The woman had been inconsolable for a year after losing him and then . . . suddenly . . . she began to experience some imperceptible discomfort in the area of the colon.

She went immediately for medical examination and was told there was nothing unusual. But she insisted on having hospital tests. The doctor complied, recognizing the source of the woman's anxiety. The tests were negative, revealing that nothing was wrong with her. She told the doctor he was stupid and found herself another doctor. She repeated the same procedure as before. Still nothing was found.

Months passed and her fear mounted. When the dye tests showed there was no cancerous tumor growing within her, she began insisting upon exploratory surgery. The doctor refused, explaining that exploratory surgery wasn't considered ethical anymore. She threatened, applied thumb screws and the doctor, no doubt seeing what was going to happen, consented to exploratory surgery.

I heard what this third doctor said to her when she was brought down from recovery. "Well, you were right, Mrs. Soanso. It's a good thing you kept after us . . . the tumor was so tiny it was barely visible to the naked eye but we got it and have prevented any further problem. You are clean as a whistle now and there is nothing more for you to worry about."

I was amazed! They found this tiny little microscopic malignancy which, I believe, hadn't been there when she first began this campaign. I saw, with revelatory light, that she had planted the seed of fear for this growth when her father became ill. She had watered it day and night with her apprehension until, finally, this tiny little thing had begun to take form in her body.

But as I saw the truth about her and the tumorous growth, the Lord gently showed me how it applied to me and the auto accident! Why, I had believed all my life . . . although I would never have put it into actual words . . . that I was going to die in a car wreck! I feared it and almost brought it upon myself.

I wonder how many times the thought, "I am afraid," stalked maliciously through my mind, churning up my emotions, affecting the functioning of my body before it brought upon me the condition I feared?

I was only twenty-five years old then, but my eyes had

been opened, by my circumstances and the guidance of the Lord, to see the way the laws governing this universe work either for or against us. If we are out of harmony with the perfect working of God's Will, conditions will prevail which are intended to bring us back into harmony. I began observing this law working in the lives of others and I saw that no one can escape the thoughts and feelings which proceed from the innermost parts.

Some thoughts and spoken words materialize almost instantly. Others may take years before they are manifested. The deciding factors are the amount of intense feeling behind the spoken word and "the fullness of time." The stronger the emotion, the quicker it will take form right before our eyes, although some decrees may not be manifested until the soul is prepared to be either blessed by a righteous decree or to learn from the consequences of an unrighteous decree.

While our words, thoughts, and emotions work as creative forces to draw the atomic building materials together in the form we have decreed, there is something else which makes it take form more certainly. That is, using the name of God to speak it into being.

When Moses encountered the burning bush in the desert, he said, " . . . *Behold, when I come unto the children of Israel, and shall say unto them, The God of your fathers hath sent me unto you; and they shall say to me, What is his name? what shall I say unto them?"* (Ex. 3:13)

"And God said unto Moses, I AM THAT I AM: and he said, thus shalt thou say unto the children of Israel, I AM hath sent me unto you." (Ex. 3:14)

Later, when the I AM THAT I AM gave the commandments to Moses to be handed down for all future generations,
He said: *"Thou shalt not take the name of the Lord thy God
in vain: for the Lord will not hold him guiltless that taketh
his name in vain."* (Ex. 20:7)

I AM THAT I AM. Was this the name by which God was
introducing Himself to His chosen people? "I AM"? That
certainly would make the name of God the unspeakable, in-
effable name, because any time I use that name I am somehow speaking for myself as well as for God. For who else can
say "I AM" for me except myself? Or who can say "I AM"
for you except yourself? And how can I speak the name
"I AM" without calling upon God Almighty, if that is the
name He has given to call upon Him?

Furthermore, He said that we are not to use His name in
vain. Was He indicating that we *could not* use His name in
vain, because whatever we decree IN HIS NAME, we would
be responsible for? And does He not say that if we vainly
used His name we would suffer the consequences? (See
Ex. 20:7)

Joel said *". . . let the weak say, I am strong."* (Joel 3:10b)
Using the name of God to decree righteousness, healing,
love, balance, deliverance has POWER FOR CREATION and
the creation will be a deliberate one, bringing about what you
desire in your heart. *"Thou shalt also decree a thing, and it
shall be established unto thee: and the light shall shine upon
thy ways."* (Job 22:28)

You can DECREE righteously in this manner: "I AM
now established in the center of God's perfect will. I AM

acting according to His direction through the Holy Spirit. As I will the Holy Spirit to live in and through me, I AM all good, I AM all love, I AM all peace; I AM all power according to His righteous and everlasting Word."

"Now faith is the substance of things hoped for, the evidence of things not seen." (Heb. 11:1) We call things which are not as though they are. Doesn't it make more sense to line up with the Word of God and start creating good and beautiful things in your world instead of the chaos and calamity you have been unwittingly setting up for yourself in the past?

In the past you have been decreeing, "I am sick." "I am tired." "I am scared." "I am no good." "I am a loser." "I am ugly." "I am fat." Even if you haven't said it aloud, you have thought it, haven't you? Every time you have thought one of these little gems, you have been sending out an unrighteous decree and have had to suffer the consequences. You have stayed just the way you decreed.

God can't be tired or weak or sick or scared or a loser. God can't be fat or dumb. Remember, *". . . the Lord will not hold him guiltless that taketh His name in vain."* (Ex. 20:7)

Most of us have the impression that "taking the name of God in vain" is using the name of God or Jesus as curse words. But when we use "I AM" to express something which God *isn't*, that is taking the name of God in vain.

We have the power to speak health or sickness to our bodies by using the name of God in a righteous decree or an unrighteous decree. And the generator of this decree is a prime target — the throat, mouth and tongue — for affliction.

Words of criticism, negativity, complaining, gossiping, lying, cursing, back-biting, talebearing and ridicule will affect the place of power within our physical bodies and eventually sap our vital energy.

BE AWARE OF WHO YOU ARE AND WHAT YOU ARE! SEE HOW MAGNIFICENTLY WE ARE MADE! We can serve God every moment of our lives, in the very spot where we are planted, if we will awaken to the reality of who and what we are and begin to use the gifts given us through the Holy Spirit!

This is growing in the fullness of Christ. It isn't just waiting until you get in a church assembly to bring forth a word of knowledge or exhortation. While this might be good, all that tremendous potential will go unused when we act like "the world."

Let's clarify "a positive decree." *It is calling things which are not as though they are.* But, *it is not calling things that are as though they are not.*

A dear friend of mine totally surprised me, recently, by going to the front of her church for "laying on of hands" for a condition of depression. Upon hearing of this, I asked if she wanted to talk about it. She said, "No." I asked why she hadn't said something about it earlier so we could pray together. She answered that she "didn't want to make a bad confession." Just two days before we had been together for Christian fellowship, and I had thought to myself, that she had never looked happier. "All a sham," she said, tearfully.

If we feel that badly, shouldn't we confess our faults one to another so that those in the "body" can pray with us and we can be healed?

Denying something which is already there is *not* a righteous decree. You cannot make something go away by saying that it isn't there. I learned this lesson the hard way!

I had been busy for weeks getting ready for a local art show, getting up early and working late in my studio. I was working through meal time, too immersed in my work to even notice hunger. I started getting a sore throat but I didn't double up on orange juice, aspirin and bed rest because I thought it was wrong to confess a sore throat, and taking "cures" would hardly have been an act of faith. "Ignore it," I told myself, "and think positive."

People are always telling new Christians . . . "Don't confess it! Claim the positive!" They tell you that whatever you confess with your mouth you are going to get. So, if you feel sickness coming on, you just stand firm and keep right on saying "I feel fine! I feel fine! I feel fine!" Even as they load your collapsed body into the ambulance and slap that oxygen mask over your face, keep right on confessing, "I feel fine!"

That sounds pretty silly but there are a lot of people doing that and also teaching others to do it. If people keep on believing that that is the way God intends for us to act, instead of seeking guidance from Him, we'll just end up with cemeteries full of good, fine, Bible-believing, faith preaching, Word-claiming, positive decreeing dead people!

The sore throat kept getting worse and worse, and before long it was so bad I could barely swallow. But I had commitments to fulfill. The day of the art show was one of those bleak November days of cold, constant rain. I got damp carrying the artwork from my car to the building, which was heated by an old-fashioned potbellied stove. I was pleased, at first, to find that my station was situated in front of the stove. But, I soon felt the disadvantages as I became over-heated and chilled as the double doors, a few feet away, were opened and closed throughout the day. By evening, my throat felt like raw meat and my voice sounded like finger-nails on a blackboard.

The autumn rain was freezing when I loaded my car with the remaining paintings at the end of the day and soon there was a coat of ice on my hair and across my shoulders. I shivered and shook all the thirty-five miles to my home. I kept confessing and affirming, "I am enjoying perfect health in Christ Jesus who has overcome sickness on my be-half. By His stripes, I am healed. My body is now manifest-ing perfect health and vitality. I am well! I am robust! I am strong! I am perfect health in His Image! Thank you, Father, in the name of Jesus!"

Two days later, I vaguely heard the six a.m. alarm sound. I struggled to get up, but fell back on the pillows into a fevered sleep. I didn't try to get up again for nearly a week. On the seventh day I struggled, with every ounce of strength I had, to get to the telephone to call a doctor. I knew I was seriously ill. I crawled to the kitchen, pulled the phone down onto the floor and croaked to the nurse, "I'm dying. Send help!"

Within twenty minutes the doctor had come to the house,

sensing there was a real emergency. He looked down my throat and gasped, "Oh, my God!" and nearly scared me over the brink. I had never heard a doctor say anything but "HMMMM" no matter how bad things were. "I must really be sick!" I thought.

My lips were so swollen and extended, I looked like a plate-mouth Ubangi. My tongue was swollen and lumpy. My throat hurt so bad I couldn't even lie down. I was propped up on several pillows. But the worst of it was the horrible, thick growth of white fuzz a quarter of an inch long which covered the entire interior of my mouth and throat and down past my larynx. The diagnosis was quinsy.

With the aid of modern medicine and the mercy of the Lord, within the month I recovered, but not without asking, over and over again, "Why, Lord? Why didn't my positive confession work? I really believed!"

When you think you have hold of something, according to the Word of God and it doesn't work, stop and find out why. Be humble before the Lord and, asking for wisdom, permit the Holy Spirit, which is the Spirit of Truth, to bring you into the understanding of the fullness of God's Word.

You see, *knowing it* and *having it* are not the same thing. So, if you pray for someone or for some situation which you are covering with a righteous decree, and you have unwavering faith in the Word of God, that He is able to deliver, and yet the answer is not manifested, ask where you are wrong. Don't wait until you end up flat on your back, like I did.

One Sunday, weeks later, while I was sitting with the choir during morning worship, the answer finally came . . . "Unless ye become as little children. . . ." That was all the Lord said, but as He spoke those words gently to my heart, the whole concept flooded my mind with new revelation.

You decree a righteous decree for that which you want to create and you confess the good, righteous, virtuous, edifying, etc.; but once something has happended to you, due to some violation of God's Law, you must become as a little child, confessing your weakness and seeking His strength and mercy. – We cannot do anything alone. The very moment we think we have the tools to bring about what we want, without relying on Him, we fall on our knees. Our Father wants us to have unquestioning faith like a little child.

When a child falls down, he runs right in and says, "Mommy, kiss it and make it better!" So Mommy kisses the boo-boo and, miraculously, the child's tears dry, a smile beams on his little face and he runs back to his play. He has faith in his parent's ability to heal his hurt.

That is the kind of faith the Father showed me I must have when I am afflicted.

On the other hand, if I had used common sense, I could have avoided that affliction. *We are living in physical bodies which will not tolerate abuse.* In fact, you have no more right to abuse your own body than you do the body of someone else. You are to care for your body as a mother nurtures the child given in her care. If you violate your responsibility, you will suffer the consequences.

According to current studies in personality and types of illnesses, each of us is prone to certain kinds of afflictions while being immune to others. I have lived in my body long enough to appraise what is necessary for my health. I know that denying my body proper rest is asking for trouble. I can go without food easier than I can go without sleep. Knowing that, I still violated my body's need by staying up late, night after night, getting ready for that art show, and lowered my body's resistance to infection.

At that time, however, I was unwisely seeing only one part of God's Word and that was the part which said not to decree unrighteousness. To treat the first signs of a growing infection would have been, I misguidedly thought, claiming an affliction for myself.

See how superstitious all this is? God has healing for us, but we have to go to Him and ask. Even Jesus had to pray to the Father in EVERYTHING in order to perform miracles.

I learned from this trying experience, a lesson of vital importance. My throat represented the place of power within me. I misused my natural power, and suffered an affliction of the throat. I forced my body past its point of endurance. The word I was using to decree a righteous decree was a misues of power, because *I was not putting my body under submission to the natural laws of health.*

The Lord revealed this to me through the account of the first miracle Jesus performed at the wedding of Cana. Cana means "place of the reeds" (in Hebrew) and the larynx is the place of the reeds (our vocal cords) within our bodies.

The wedding at Cana represented a symbolical marriage of the soul and body working together in spiritual union. The changing of the water into wine represented the changed condition which takes place in us when we are decreeing under the power of the Holy Spirit. When the Spirit is operative in us and we are aligned with the Word of God, body, soul and spirit, we can and frequently do speak conditions into existence. Once we become aware of this power within us, we need to carefully weigh what we say and the manner in which we say it. *"Let your speech be alway with grace, seasoned with salt, that ye may know how ye ought to answer every man."* (Col. 4:6)

Seeing the weight of the spoken word, sixteen years ago, through this affliction, I prayed to be able always to consecrate my words and my voice unto Him so that I could speak the Word of life and hope to others. I fail more often than I care to admit, because the tongue is the hardest member of the body to train. But the Lord is patient and the Holy Spirit is my inner witness. When I fail, He brings all things to remembrance so that I can ask forgiveness. But, oh the joy when He adds His power to my spoken word, enabling me to speak "Peace!" with divine authority. In my work with the handicapped, retarded, mentally ill, and those sick unto death, I know when I am "sounding brass" and when God has placed the power of love behind my spoken words. My words alone can do nothing but my words with His power can set people free!

Not long ago, I was privileged to use my consecrated words to talk an old blind man into the next world. I loved this dear old soul and cared for him in his last days as a mother would care for an infant. He was so pitifully helpless.

Coming from Scotland, he had few close relatives in this country. His wife, Mary, had preceded him in death and he had no children. He was frightened, toward the end, when the blackness of death became darker than the blackness of his blindness. I stayed by his side, holding his gnarled old hand and talked to him until he breathed his last breath.

We talked about the journey ahead and what was in store for him on the other side. I guided him to look for the light of Christ, for whosoever seeks, shall find. I told him how to open his spiritual eyes to see the world into which he was going. I encouraged him to concentrate upon that world and forget about this one. I told him that, as he used his spiritual eyes to look into the next world, he would soon see someone who would lead him into the new world and that when he saw the Light of Glory, he would know that he was on the right path.

I could tell him these things because I believe them with every part of my being. I have seen many people "die" and depart from this world. Those who know the Lord depart in peace and glory.

When I paused, momentarily, to wipe away the tears which were overcoming me, he quickly said in his thick Scottish brogue, "Oh, doon stop tawking now, Joo-ice! Y'make alll the fearrr g'way with yerrr swit voo-ice."

His clear blue eyes were brightly sparkling and his ruddy face was aglow with the anticipation of what was just ahead. All fear had left him. Suddenly, he called out, "Mary, Mary! Y'dinna forget me!" and with a sigh, he just stepped clear of that ancient worn out body. There was a beautiful look of joy and peace on his face, and I could visualize Thomas and Mary with all vestiges of age and sickness gone, walking through sunlit fields of heather on their way home.

I was still holding his work-worn hand as I whispered, "God speed, Thomas! See you at the Throne!" and for awhile, I just sat there alone in his dim room, feeling the supernatural power who had been summoned to receive another soul into glory.

It wasn't until later that I realized that while the words we speak are vitally important, it is even more important to have our voices dedicated to His use so that the Spirit is able to speak just the right words for every situation. And somehow, not because of me, but in spite of me, the Holy Spirit was able to say "*. . . my peace give I unto you: not as the world giveth, give I unto you . . .* " (John 14:27) *"Lord, now lettest thou thy servant depart in peace, according to thy Word: . . . "* (Luke 2:29)

7

"Forgive...And Be Healed."

"And be ye kind one to another, tenderhearted, forgiving one another, even as God for Christ's sake hath forgiven you." (Eph. 4:32)

There is no other state of mind which can cause more sickness and physical distress than unforgiveness. Unforgiveness eats away at the physical body in the same manner that acid can destroy the container in which it is stored. Unforgiveness, with its partners of destruction, resentment and revenge, can destroy the soul, poison our social lives, thwart our careers and even cause mental illness. Unforgiveness is one of the most serious sins we can commit.

Sin separates us from God. Sin cuts off God's flow of blessings to us. We don't pray when we are in sin. We don't feel the presence of the Holy Spirit. We don't permit Him to work through us. Sin makes us ashamed and causes us to hide from the face of God.

Unforgiveness causes us to sit in on judgement on another human being. We determine that they do not deserve our

forgiveness, that what they did was too horrible to be forgiven . . . and that is judgement. *"Judge not, that ye be not
judged. For with what judgement ye judge, ye shall be judged:
and with what measure ye mete, it shall be measured to you
again."* (Matt. 7:1-2)

We cannot judge another without being judged ourselves.
If we determine that another person is unwarranting forgiveness we are proclaiming that exact same judgement upon
ourselves. It is not merely a poetic pronouncement on "how
to win friends and influence people." The very Son of God
came down from glory with living words of spirit and said to
us, *"Don't judge other people or you will be judged. And
whatever you do to others, the same thing is going to come
upon you."* (Matt. 7:1 Paraphrased) This is a law! A cosmic,
divine, absolute, spiritual law. And the laws of God are not
subject to revision, eradication or alteration. They are eternal,
impersonal, impartial cosmic laws which are no respecter of
persons.

So many times, when encountering the laws of God or the
cosmic laws of the universe (which is saying exactly the same
thing, for this world is the Lord's and all that is in it) we find
that, although the receiver of the law tactfully engraved
the stones with THOU SHALT NOT, the truth is WE DARE
NOT act in violation or avoidance of God's laws. We may try.
But we don't get away with it. Because whatsoever we mete
out to someone else, it is measured again unto us.

The ideal prayer model which Jesus gave us in *The Lord's
Prayer* (Matt. 6:9-13) teaches us unnullifiable truth of *Divine
Ordinance* . . . as you do unto others it shall be done unto

you. There is no salvation without forgiveness of sins and there is no forgiveness of our sins unless we be willing to relinquish unforgiveness in our hearts toward those who have sinned against us. The forgiveness we seek is measured out to us in exact proportion to the forgiveness we give others. *And forgive us our debts, as we forgive our debtors.* Each time we repeat *The Lord's Prayer* we are, in effect, reestablishing our relationship with our Father. We are saying, "Yes, I understand and I agree. You don't have to forgive me one bit more than I am willing to forgive those who have hurt me."

Judgement of another requires gross conceit on our part. By what do we judge, except by our own standards? We are, in effect, saying, "This is the way that I do things and, of course, you know that I am always right. You should do things the same way I do them, and if you don't I won't be able to forgive you." We say, "I am slender and I think you should be slender, too." Or "I don't think you should drink alcoholic beverages because I don't."

Most of us don't always make these judgements aloud. Like the cowards that all unrighteous judges are, we hide behind a facade of excuses which sound much more compassionate . . . but the effects are the same. We have determined, according to our own choices, what another should do with the free will God gave him. We have determined that he or she should use that free will to be like us. Have you any idea how much misery comes into your life by making such judgements? Every time you are confronted with a person or situation which isn't to your specifications you be-

come upset or angry. The judgement begins the cankerous
work of unforgiveness in your heart. Truthfully, you are
trying to control the lives of others. None of us has that
right. We are accountable to God *only* for the choices *we*
make. We can't make determinations for the lives of others.
We can only make them for ourselves.

Just as the rich soil beyond our window must be cul-
tivated for the seeds which shall be planted, so our minds
have to be prepared to receive seeds of disharmony and
discord. If we don't prepare the soil of our minds the seeds
can't produce roots and grow. Instead of allowing judgement
to form say, "In the name of Jesus Christ, I bless you this
day with His Love as it flows forth from my spirit!" – That's
powerful! That is taking command of your mind and not
allowing the enemy to use you to express his hatred and
contempt for God's beautiful creation. Since the mind is
not a void which can be empty of thought, I desire to put
into my mind what *I* want there, not what the enemy wants
there. *"Thy Word has entered into my heart that I might not
sin against thee."* (Psa. 119:11 Paraphrased)

All judgements are not fleeting determinations made upon
strangers or acquaintances. Most of us have several judgements which were made at a time past when someone has
wronged us, and we have seen no reason to change our
opinions of that person. We have brought them before our
court of justice, and as judge, jury, and prosecuting attorney,
we have found them guilty, – judgement unanimously passed.
We have announced, "no mercy," and handed down a life
sentence. But what we have not recognized in these inter-

vening years is that, while that person has been in the prison of our hearts, we have had to stand guard at the cell door. Perhaps it was because we found the offender to be such a dangerous criminal and felt it necessary to have him shackled to us. But how free can one be with another chained to his arm? Has he been able to forget that person even for a moment? Has he had freedom to enjoy life while guarding a prisoner chained in his dingy jail?

It has been my observation, as I have "sat by the highway" and studied life, that there is little difference in consciousness between the sick and those who tend the sick; between the mentally ill and those who guard them; between the criminal and the prison guard. We are all attracted to a certain station in life, according to the level of consciousness we possess, and it takes two poles of the same force for that energy to be activated. Just as sadists and masochists tend to marry each other, the jailor and the jailed are usually only a cell door apart.

And so the unforgiveness we have bound to ourselves keeps the pain of the transgression alive. Some say, "Well, I can forgive but I can't forget." That is not true. If we can't — we are unwilling to forget, and thus, we haven't forgiven.

Remembering means to put together again . . . putting the "members" of something or someone back together. If what you are re-membering is the painful transgressions of another toward you, you are mentally recreating the experience. It is as though you have the words "THIS IS A REENACTMENT" flashed on your mental "screen": You are wired with electrodes to one of the machines used in a hospital. During the re-membering your blood pressure has become exhilarated, your pulse and heart beat quickened, the flow of adrenalin is increased, the oxygen level of your blood depreciates as your breathing becomes rapid and shallow, and your blood vessels are constricted. It is as though the experience is taking place at this precise moment.

Remembering involves looking into the past. Lot's wife looked back after she had been told not to look back. As she got to the edge of those condemned cities she heard the flames crackling through the timbers of the burning buildings, the screams of people meeting their cataclysmic death, the hissing of water streams as they heated to boiling, and the horrible thuds of stone falling upon stone. She looked back. And when she did, she turned into a pillar of salt.

There is a valuable lesson to be learned here. Some have interpreted it to mean that God didn't want her longing after the sins for which the city was known, and her looking back meant she wasn't ready to give up the sin life in order to enter into a life of spiritual sanctification. The lesson hidden here applies to everyone of us . . . for some of us have not had such a clear-cut decision required of us. Some of us have been Christians all our lives and yet have intensified our walk in a gradual manner. We, too, have stood where Lot's wife stood.

Food preservation has always been a concern to man. In Lot's time there was no refrigeration. In a land of such intense desert clime, it must have been even more difficult for them to preserve food from spoiling. The method of saving foods from one season to another was limited to drying and salting. Figs and dates and grapes were dried while olives and fish were salted. Lot's wife, also, was preserved in salt because of her looking back.

Our unforgiveness is a looking back process, and by doing this, we *preserve* the memory within us, . . . just as a pillar of salt. And that pillar of salt is visible to God. He looks into our hidden recesses and sees that the pillar of salt is still there. Perhaps it looks like a statue of someone we have not forgiven.

As long as that "pillar of salt" is within us we can't have complete salvation. Salvation is for every sinner who confesses his sins and has them forgiven. Jesus Christ, through an act of grace and love, came to earth to bring SALVATION to man. He is the *Ideal, Supreme Perfection* in *embodiment* form. He is The Lord of lords, and King of kings. There is none other. He is Perfection personified. He said, *"Forgive us our debts, as we forgive our debtors . . . "* (Matt. 6:12), and: *" . . . I am the way, the truth and the life: no man cometh unto the Father, but by me."* (John 14:6) *"Remember therefore from whence thou art fallen, and repent, and do the first works; or else I will come unto thee quickly, and will remove thy candlestick from out of his place, except thou repent."* (Rev. 2:5) *"If we confess our sins, he is faithful and just to forgive our sins, and to cleanse us from all unrighteousness."* (John 1:9) *"Draw nigh to God, and He will draw nigh to you. Cleanse your hands, ye sinners; and purify your hearts, ye double-minded. Be afflicted, and mourn, and weep: let your laughter be turned to mourning, and your joy to heaviness. Humble yourselves in the sight of the Lord and he shall lift you up."* (James 4:8-10)

We are living in the latter days. The Lord is calling us to come into the Holy Place but we cannot go until we are prepared. We have to be clean — clean on the inside which will make us clean all over. Remember, unforgiveness is the main iniquity which is holding back the Body of Christ. As long as our eyes are fixed upon Jesus, Son of Glory, what happens to us at the hands of another person cannot take root in our hearts. When we take our eyes off Jesus, we might be doing so because we want to "fight it out" with this person. Then, we are creating a situation which is triple-fold: we make it difficult to forgive him, we make it difficult for him to forgive us, and we make it difficult to forgive ourselves.

If we lose the battle it is because we agreed in our minds, beforehand, that we were going to go down to Satan's level and let him make fools of us. One of the main reasons we continue to lose the battle when power and principalities come against us is because of the deadly sin of self-indulgence . . . SELF PITY.

Self-pity is a deadly sin because it opens the door to the realm of darkness. All the demons of hell can come rushing in against us when we start that "poor little me" routine.

Thoughts such as, "Why me, Lord?" begin to crowd the consciousness instead of "The Lord is my defense; and my God is the rock of my refuge." With self-pity comes doubt and wavering faith in His Perfect Will. If we had held fast to the vision of our Lord Triumphant and claimed our victory through Him the attack would have ended as soon as we cried, *"Lord, my foot slippeth!"* (See Psa. 94:18)

Self-pity is emotional wallowing in tears. It is easy for Satan to turn our minds when we reveal this "chink in our armour." We have already allowed him to come in the moment we turned our eyes away from Jesus and to ourselves. As long as we remain in self-pity our ears are tuned to hear every single word Satan whispers. And if we listen to what he says he will destroy us.

He will influence our thinking until we agree with him and become convinced that, "No one cares what happens to me. I'm not appreciated around here at all. No matter what I do, it never makes any difference. Why should I try so hard? Who cares? I'm no good. I am worthless. I probably deserve the treatment I am getting. No sense in going on. No one will miss me. They'll probably be glad I'm gone. What good has it done me to try to live a good life? Am I being blessed? Is this my reward?" When we start thinking along these lines, Satan says to his henchmen, "We got him now, fellas! Reel him in!" Satan's work is easy after that. We are like "silly putty" in his hands. We might attempt suicide, while in such a mental state, and end up in psychiatric ward. We won't even remember that it all started with self-pity!

Self-pity results in a distortion of every truth we have ever known. It is as though the lens of our eyes have been warped so that everything we look at is like the images in mirrors in a fun house. We have been given a delusion and if we persist, we will believe a lie.

Realizing that we are responsible for the Satanic attack we have received at the hands of those about us, we should take responsibility for our state of mind. We should stay away from the door which leads to darkness and refuse to allow self-pity to begin. As we take responsibility for the prevention of future attacks, we must recognize the part we have played in the attacks of the past . . . those very attacks supervised by the people whom we have found so hard to forgive. Knowing the truth of all things really does set us free!

Jesus said, *"Enter ye in at the strait gate: for wide is the gate, and broad is the way, that leadeth to destruction, and many there be which go in thereat: Because strait is the gate, and narrow is the way, which leadeth unto life, and few there be that find it."* (Matt. 7:13-14)

The doorway into the enemy's world is understandably wide and easily accessible. That is why so many people enter without resistance. They do not take control of their thoughts. They allow the mind to run unfettered and it . . . like all things . . . will follow the path of least resistance. The currents of an uncontrolled mind are swift, and, if not prevented, can carry us into subterranean stratum of the dark side of our minds where we may have great difficulty finding the way back.

But God has given us dominion over all things! If we used the ability God has placed in man we would not only have dominion over the herb, the mineral and all the animals, but also over the forces of the winds, the sun, the waters, and the forces within man. The priority, of course, is to subdue the thoughts spawned by our own minds. Until we do that, we will forever struggle under the whim of circumstance and we will never be what God intended us to be.

We have been inundated with darkness for such a long time that we have begun to believe in the shadows reflected on the walls of our inner caves. It is written, *"The people which sat in darkness saw great light; and to them which sat in the region and shadow of death light is sprung up."* (Matt. 4:16) And again, it is written, *"And this is the condemnation, that light is come into the world, and men loved darkness rather than light, because their deeds were evil. For every one that doeth evil hateth the light, neither cometh to the light, lest his deeds should be reproved. But he that doeth truth cometh to the light, that his deeds may be made manifest, that they are wrought in God."* (John 3:19-21)

Obviously, that means that it is possible to have victory over darkness. It is possible to forgive so that we may be forgiven. We have never been asked to do something which cannot or has never been done.

We need a change in consciousness in order to successfully resist the irresistible pull of the negative forces of darkness seeking to bring us into the "lower kingdom." It isn't easy. If it were we would all have become "as the gods," needing neither salvation nor grace. But, though we rise and fall, rise again only to fall again, we never fall quite so far as we did the time before, nor as low as we did before He found us. Our awareness of our utter dependency upon Him grows and, as it does, the more we give Him the rightful place in our consciousness. When we allow Him to occupy the throne within our hearts, we discover, for ourselves, that He will assist us in breaking old mental habits, and help us fight the negativity within. But, it is still up to us to keep constant vigilance over our thoughts. And it is our responsibility to wear the armour of God AT ALL TIMES.

It is incredible that we have been given this spiritual armour to protect us and we leave it lying around in some closet where it never does us any good. Some who wear the armour "in public" make the mistake of taking it off as soon as they get home. The enemy is no dummy. If he wants to get to us, what better way than through someone we love and trust? I have seen Satanic attacks where the person changes so fast from being himself or herself to something so ugly that I have wanted to run and hide. I have seen faces change where one would hardly know it was the same person. And it has always been because SATAN wanted to stop spiritual growth. It was never because that person wanted to stop it. — See who it is who is coming against you and do battle " . . . *against principalities, against powers, against the rulers of the darkness of this world, against spiritual wickedness in high places."* (Eph. 6:12) Take authority over the situation in the name of Jesus. And physically move through the entire area, claiming it all in the name of Jesus. Rebuke any influence which is not of God. And peace will be restored. And the incident forgotten. And love will continue. Because that is what God wants, that is what you want and that is what the enemy can't stand!

Once you see the truth of a situation in the Light shed upon your life by Christ, you know *you can* pull every spiritual tool you have to fight for right and that as a child of God, you should. But if you get mired down at the level of the world you won't settle anything. You will just make matters worse and a lot of people will get hurt.

Don't you suppose that the person attacking you is just as miserable as you are? Don't you suppose that somewhere deep down inside he would like to have the hate and meanness expunged from his soul so he can stop using all his energy to hurt you? I am convinced that this is true. There are so many testimonies of hardened criminals, *Hell's Angels, Mafia* members, *KKK* leaders, *Black Panthers, acid rock stars,* and *prisoners* on death row who have been touched by the loving hand of Jesus Christ and are now converted. I am convinced that everyone wants to be good and loving and kind. They want to have that joy which springs up from inside in rivers of living water but they don't know how to get it and they don't realize that Satan has a hold on their heartstrings, keeping them all tied up inside with resentment, insecurity and unforgiveness.

That should enable us to forgive those who trespass against us. We know that Satan is a murderer and a liar and a thief. He is gambling for high stakes . . . the souls of mankind which Jesus has bought with His precious blood . . . and he will go to any lengths to steal away the souls of the people around you. You know that without the influence of Satan working through these people that they are lovable, not only to God, but to you. You have loved them in the past and can love them again. You can be friends again or lovers or family.

Ask the Father to give you a forgiving heart. Ask in faith, believing in the name of Jesus that whatsoever you ask it shall be given to you. Ask not only to forgive but to forget and never call to mind again the hurts that have been done to

you. Ask the Father now in the name of Jesus to heal you on
the inside, way deep down in your soul and then know that it
is His pleasure to give you all good things because He loves
you. Know that this is the basis for all the healing you
are ever going to need in the future. Once you allow the
Father to work in you, in this manner, you will find that
you are given new life and one more abundant than you
ever had before. If you have sincerely prayed for this healing
of the inner man, know that your prayer has been heard
and it is done. You are now on the way to *New Life, New
You,* and *New Health!*

Now don't spoil what has just been done by the Love of
the Father by saying, "But I didn't feel like anything happened!" I once made the mistake of thinking that when I
prayed for something I would have to have some kind of
experience to let me know that my prayer had been answered.
You know, like the earth moving or lightning striking or at
least being overcome by a brilliant light. Something profound
that would let me know, beyond a shadow of a doubt, that
the Lord had heard and answered. Sometimes it happens like
that. Most of the time, it doesn't. I prayed to forgive the person who had done so much to hurt me but I didn't get any
feeling, whatsoever, that my prayer had been answered. The
next time I encountered that person, I got all those same old
jumpy feelings in my stomach, my hands began to perspire
and my knees got shaky. So I said to myself, "Well, the Lord
hasn't answered my prayer yet. I haven't gotten over all
those bad feelings I have had so I must not have really forgiven her." And then I would worry over it because I knew

what the Word said about forgiveness. I had head knowledge
. . . but not enough to make me wise.

I knew I had to forgive in order to be forgiven. If I wasn't
forgiven how was I going to get into heaven? So I would go
back to pray some more and plead and cry and beg the
Father to give me a forgiving heart so I could get over all that
horrible condition which was eating away at me.

But it just never went away and I never got the feeling that
I had been given the forgiving heart that I wanted and needed.
I went to a *Kathryn Kuhlman* service one Good Friday in
Pittsburgh. I went to be healed of unforgiveness. I wanted
more than anything in the whole world to have the experi-
ence of forgiveness toward that person. Every time that per-
son's name was mentioned, my jaws would tighten up and
I would start shaking.

Forgiveness isn't a feeling. It is a *decision* we make or refuse to make. It is a cool, calculated, rational, mental decision. If we decide in our hearts that we want to forgive someone because we love Jesus and don't want anything to separate us from Him, then it is done!

By the same token, when we say we can't forgive that
person, what we're really saying is: "Jesus, I have made the
decision not to forgive. I don't want to!" And, we can make
a decision to not forgive ourselves.

I wanted to forgive, and if I had known that the decision
I made to forgive was the beginning of the working of righteousness within me I could have been spared the misery I
suffered. But, perhaps I wouldn't have learned the lesson so
well. I learned that, if we pray, asking whatsoever we will in

the name of Jesus, and if we have the Word in us, as He is the Word, then we must have faith that He will be faithful to give us whatsoever we ask. We must believe that. We can't analyze it, dissect it, measure it, prove it, or debate it. It is so. And in faith, we believe. He wants us to have life abundant and He has made every provision for us to have it. Garbing ourselves in sackcloth and ashes over a past sin which we can't forget is not only foolishness, it is tantamount to spiritual pride.

I know about spiritual pride. Once I thought I was so righteous! How many times I said that I had walked the "higher road" since I was four years old. I walked on a chalk line. I said to people who wanted me to do "worldly things" with them that I would rather be alone with all the world against me than to do something which would displease Him. I said, "Jesus and I are a majority." I said I didn't care what the world did or how the mores changed, there was only one Truth and that is what has been handed down by God. And I said those things when I was just a little tot and when I was a teen-ager and when I was an airline stewardess and when I became a mother. I said it in an impassioned sermon when I was nine years old; I said it to a group of college friends at a New Year's Eve party, I said it to a government official who was my high superior and held the future of my career in his hands, and I said it to my employer.

A woman in one of my Bible Study classes asked me, one night, "What would you do if you did such and such?" and I answered. "Oh, but I wouldn't." She said, "But what if . . . " And I said, "I wouldn't!" And she said, "But what if you just fell into temptation and it got too much for you to resist?" And I said, "It wouldn't happen! I know myself!"

It is written, *"For by thy words thou shalt be justified, and by thy words thou shalt be condemned."* (Matt. 12:37) Never think there is something you wouldn't do. That is spiritual pride. And pride goeth before the fall!

But following repentance there is sweet redemption. It is never so sweet as when we need it personally. When there is a breaking of the spirit of pride and the molding of a contrite heart the precious robe of humility is laid upon your shoulders, and, you see then how foolish you were to boast anything of yourself, for the greatest thing we have is but a filthy rag before His righteousness. And we know, from the depths of our souls, that we would gladly shed blood to receive forgiveness for our sins so that we may share glory with Him forever and ever. And then we see Him there, reaching down to us into our self-made pit of destruction with His nail-pierced hands and for the very first time in our lives we realize that we have caused that wound upon His perfect body. That is when we know, Oh Lord, how we now know, that all the blood that was needed to wash away those sins has already been shed and we are forgiven. Can we, in the light of His endless mercy do anything else but forgive?

8

The Endless Struggle.

Beyond the resplendance of the cosmos, the intricacies of multiple universes, the priceless value of untold treasuries of mineral wealth, the unmatched beauty of the varied faces of this planet, the limitless magnificence of the heavens, the majesty of the countless untamed beasts, birds and multiple-colored fishes, man is the crowning glory of it all!

How we can marvel at the stupendous reality of that truth when we look at mankind from our lateral position. *"Thou madest him a little lower than the angels; thou crownedst him with glory and honor, and didst set him over the works of thy hands: thou hast put all things in subjection under his feet."* (Heb. 2:7)

The possibilities which God has designed for man are beyond our wildest dreams or expectations, because we do not even perceive what we are. Yet, in spite of our ignorance of self, there is within man the irrepressible urge to know God; the form seeking to know the Formless who formed him. We look toward the heavens with a sense of awe, oblivious to the fact that the manifested form of creation and its relationship to the Creator is the macrocosmic pattern of physical man and his relationship to his spirit. We know that whatever truth we perceive of God is applicable to ourselves because man is created in the Image of God and in His Likeness.

God is Spirit; man is spirit. God is manifested in His creation; man is manifested in the physical body. God has expressed Himself in the person of Christ, Mediator between heaven and earth; between God and man. And even as Christ marks that point between the invisible Spirit of God and His visible creation, the soul of man marks the point between the invisible spirit and the physical.

"And the Lord God formed man of the dust of the ground, and breathed into his nostrils the breath of life; (pneuma, Greek: spirit) *and man became a living soul."* (Gen. 2:7)

The breath of life which God breathed into Adam-man was an exhalation of His own Spirit substance so that although man would have individualized egos developing according to his experience on earth, there would remain that controlling force in man which would originate in God, without beginning and without end.

Adam-man was therefore created by God, an archetypal pattern for all mankind, and he was all of what we term spirit, soul, intellect, and body. Adam was physical man, raised up out of the elements of this planet and the first motion of individualized mind in contact with and animating substance. Although the Adam-ego could identify with the material form, it was also in a state of spiritual illumination. Adam was *aware* of God!

It was this perfect rapport with the mind of God which made Adam's world a paradise. That first man had *God-consciousness*. In our fallen state, *God-consciousness has been replaced with faith*. We hope for things unseen. But the original state of man was the ability to see the things for which he hoped. His consciousness adhered perfectly to the wisdom and perfection of God.

Adam was the first created spirit-man. We know that this is the form of the original creation because he was made in the Image and Likeness of God and God is Spirit. *"And the Lord God caused a deep sleep to fall upon Adam, and he slept: and he took one of his ribs, and closed up the flesh instead thereof: And the rib, which the Lord God had taken from man, made he a woman, and brought her unto the man."* (Gen. 2:21)

The Bible is a fantastic work beyond the greatest genius of man, because not only does it give us historical account of our heritage from our earth parents, but also tells us, in symbolical form, the spiritual heritage we have from our Father-Creator.

Adam was given a help-meet whom he named "Eve, because she was the mother of all living." This information is important to us at two levels. Historically, Adam and Eve are the parents of all living people on Earth. Symbolically, they are even more important to us in the understanding of our nature.

From Adam, spirit-man living in a body made of the elements of the earth, was made Eve, his help-meet whose name means "elementary life" or "luminous elementary life."

Eve represents the feminine aspect of the generic man, the part of his individualized consciousness which is the feeling or emotional aspect. The tradition that Eve was made from a rib over Adam's heart further indicates a specific emotion . . . that of love. Further, the heart was considered the seat of the soul so, in actuality, Eve is representative of the soul of Adam-man.

The Hebrew verb, "hoh," which is the basis of "Eve" also forms the basis of the name Jehovah so we see that there is a similarity of purpose or origin. However, in referring to "Eve" there is a slight change in characters and a hardening of the vowels so that it no longer represents absolute life as does "hoh." The root meaning of "Eve" becomes "the struggle of elementary life." This indicates the struggle which the soul encounters in its attempt to regain its perfect state of existence which it held with the Absolute God before falling into a state of duality. It is this perpetual struggle of the soul for dominance over the flesh that will be discussed in this chapter.

From almost the beginning of time, records and hieroglyphics indicate that man has awareness of and belief in his eternal soul. In some cultures it was regarded as the motivating force behind man's life. Ancient and traditional beliefs have frequently portrayed the soul in symbolical terms as the virgin madonna who lovingly and sacrificially cared for her infant child, a representative of the mortal self.

Biblical symbology has named the soul "the bright morning star," the "day star" and in several Scriptures, the soul of an individual was called "his angel," as indicated in these

Scriptures:

"We have also a more sure word of prophecy; whereunto ye do well that ye take heed, as unto a light that shineth in a dark place, until the day dawn, and the day star arise in your hearts: . . . " (2 Pet. 1:19)

" . . . when the morning stars sang together, and all the sons of God shouted for joy?" (Job 38:7)

"Take heed that ye despise not one of these little ones; for I say unto you, That in heaven their angels do always behold the face of my Father which is in heaven." (Matt. 18:10)

"For the Sadducees say that there is no resurrection, neither angel, nor spirit: but the Pharisees confess both." (Acts 23:8)

The soul of an individual may make its presence felt in a dream as the "shadow" which stands at the right side just out of the dreamer's view. The benevolent feeling projected from the soul gives the dreamer a feeling of protection and love. Or a person may see a vision or reveries where the soul is depicted as an angel possessing all wisdom and power. Each of these symbolic presentations however, bears one common description of the soul; the soul is older, wiser, stronger, more powerful, more righteous than the human self and acts as an advocate or messenger of God.

This theme is prevalent in every religion and among every people on this planet. Man, created in the Image of God, as spirit, has a soul which indwells the mortal body of flesh and that luminous absolute life has different degrees of awareness through which it functions.

The soul is in a state of perpetual growth in its struggle to return to its perfect Edenic state. The struggle in which mortal man is engaged with the forces of light and darkness attains for him a measure of wisdom which is assimilated by the soul and aids it in its growth. The outcome of this dualistic conflict will be its completed Image of God in manifested form with a spirit which is self-aware as well as God-conscious. The soul will then have eliminated all delusion of separation from the Creator and all dualistic thoughts of negativity and darkness will be done away. Clothed in "robes of righteousness," the soul will then have a body which has been changed from the corruptible to the incorruptible, from perishable to imperishable. We shall then be made "whole."

We are not "whole" at present. Nor have we been since the Adamic fall. We are so accustomed to our fragmentation, however, that we do not even think we are unusual or abnormal. But, what great and glorious things He has in store for us. *"For God, who commanded the light to shine out of darkness, hath shined in our hearts, to give the light of the knowledge of the glory of God in the face of Jesus Christ. But we have this treasure in earthen vessels, . . . for which cause we faint not; but though our outward man perish, yet the inward man is renewed day by day."* (2 Cor. 4:6-7, 16)

The inward man is the soul. The soul is the entirety of man's consciousness; that which he has appropriated both from the mortal mind's knowledge and experience and from the cognizant wisdom from the spirit. The soul is both conscious and subconscious. It is in the realm of the soul that all ideas begin to take form. The soul is not the realm of God mind but rather a diffusion of God mind, a second emanation even as the Garden of Eden was a second emanation of heaven. Just as Eden was given to man as a perfect dwelling place where he could meet with and commune with his Creator, so is the soul. This is the place of all divine possibilities, once we turn to the side of light within the soul and away from the side of darkness. *"To open their eyes, and to turn them from darkness to light, and from the power of Satan unto God, . . . "* (Acts 26:18) *"For ye were sometimes darkness, but now are ye light in the Lord: walk as children of light: . . . Wherefore he saith, Awake thou that sleepest, and arise from the dead, and Christ shall give thee light."* (Eph. 5:8, 14) *"Then shall thy light break forth as the morning, and thine health shall spring forth speedily: and thy righteousness shall go before thee; the glory of the Lord shall be thy reward."* (Isa. 58:8)

The Garden of Eden also signifies the soul's worship of the one true God. As long as man recognizes and honors only God, he dwells in a realm of perfect harmony and peace. This is a state of consciousness which can make any physical place an "Eden." But once the mind is divided between good and evil, man is driven out of "Eden" and forced to suffer the consequences of eating that bitter fruit of "the knowledge of good and evil" all the days of his life, or until he becomes aware that his sorrow is the result of the dualistic thought processes.

There are many accounts in the Bible which allegorically capture, for our enlightenment, the grand work of the soul. The stories are actual historical accounts of real people and real happenings. But the hand of God is in these anecdotes so that they are meaningful to all people of all ages, who are at different levels of awareness and spiritual insight. The story of Josiah, a king of Judah, is an example:

The name "Josiah" means in Hebrew *fire of Jehovah.* Fire is symbolic of power of the spirit. "Josiah" also is interpreted "whom Jehovah supports" or "whom Jehovah heals." The story of Josiah graphically and symbolically explains how we are to: *"Labor not for the meat which perisheth, but for that meat which endureth unto everlasting life, which the Son of man shall give unto you: . . . "* (John 6:27)

When Josiah began his reign over Judah, the children of God were again idol worshipping. Because of sense identification, they were constantly slipping away from the worship of the one true God. The story of Israel is the story of mankind, for we are all in such a state and continually are falling away to the worship of false gods. Every time we permit the faculties of mind to determine truth for us, every time we are drawn to some material thing because of the predominating desire of the senses, we are, in effect, falling away unto false gods. We give ourselves over to sense consciousness instead of spiritual consciousness and thus, we are not able to worship God in truth. It is only through the spirit that we are able to worship God in truth.

Josiah ordered a purging of Judah and Jerusalem. All idols were to be removed from the temple, and the bones of dead priests were ordered dug up and burned in order that they could not be revered by the worshippers. Josiah was only a child . . . a mere eight years old . . . when this work began.

This symbolizes that when we are "baby Christians," there

is a certain cleansing of the temple which must take place, and of course, the body is our temple. Remember, we were idol worshippers when we were in the world so there is a lot of debris in our temples which must be cleansed.

Initially, this cleansing will be the elimination of those sense habits which have kept us in bondage to the flesh. Some converts are immediately cleansed of such unworthy behavior while others persist in some habit of the flesh.

Following such outward sense attachments there is a cleansing which involves the discipline of training the mind to think on positive, good, clean, virtuous things, and a systematic denial of error thoughts which have become habitual in both the objective and the subjective consciousness. Error thoughts include the thought of evil, the power of Satan, the bondage of poverty, sickness, depression and any other, *". . . imagination and high thing which exalteth itself against the knowledge of God . . . "* (2 Cor. 10:5)

Immediately following this purging of consciousness, the builders of the land (2 Kings 2) must be put to work to restore the temple. These "builders" are positive decrees which we use to establish righteousness in the temple. We have to fill the void left by eliminating negative thought patterns, or else the mind would quickly be filled with other negative or harmful thoughts.

All this work is begun at the conscious level of man's awareness and requires constant discipline. The moment we relax in our prayer life and reading of the Word the darkness of negativity springs up in us. It is still there at the subconscious level, due to the years of practice we have had

in thinking as the world thinks — the profanity, the off-
color jokes, the lust of the eye. But discipline is functional
at the conscious level for only awhile. Eventually, due to
habit once again, the mind needs to be emptied to learn
new skills, to absorb the Word of God, and finally, thoughts
which are occupying the consciousness are delegated to the
subconsciousness.

As an example of this process, consider your learning how
to drive an automobile. It was such a complicated effort,
having to think of so many things at once and watch in so
many directions all at the same time. Now that you're more
experienced, you can drive for hundreds of miles and not be
consciously occupied with the speedometer or the mechanics
of piloting that car. You are able to listen to the radio, eat a
sandwich, carry on a conversation, observe the route markers
and road signs, the cars beside, before and behind you and
maneuver the car, all at the same time. You can do that
because everything you learned about driving is programmed
into the subconscious mind now and can be done while the
conscious mind is considering new thoughts.

So it is with the training of the wholeness of man into the
fullness of Christ. In 2 Chron. 34:14-28, we read that when
Josiah was king of Judah, the book of the law was found in
the temple. Because "Josiah" means "whom Jehovah heals"
we see a symbolical representation of the spiritually awakened individual who seeks to do the will of God, but first
needs healing or forgiveness in order to carry out his desire.

The book of law which was found in the House of God
represents the truth that in the spiritual consciousness of

man, the law of God is written, so that all men, whether
they be worshippers of false gods or whether they be actively
engaged in seeking out the one true God, have equal opportunity to receive the fullness of God's blessing through His
revelation of Himself. As Josiah discovers this book of law,
he receives the truth of God's Word and rents his garments
in sorrow that he had not known beforehand the admonition
concerning the law which had been laid out for the children
of Israel. This is the moment of conversion both for Josiah
and for us when all false beliefs are torn away by the truth
of God's Word, and true repentance for past sins humble us
before the Almighty mercy of God.

When God's law is revealed to us, the subconscious powers
of the soul are brought into activity which aid us in attaining
that which God has decreed. The impression of the glories of
God begin to shine into the dark recesses of the soul so that
man wants to consecrate himself to his Maker and to begin
to use the powers of his mortal mind, plus the strength of the
physical body, to bring about the restoration of the temple.

The revelatory faculty of the soul is brought about through
the love nature, the "Eve, mother of all living things" part of
the individual. This is the new heart and the new mind which
is given at conversion. With the feeling nature now spiritualized, man becomes tender-hearted and nonresistant toward
the call of God. He is now born into God's kingdom at this
point and no longer leans toward the carnal call of the world.

And now the regenerative work can begin for the way
has been opened for the fire of the Holy Spirit. *"And Josiah
took away all the abominations out of all the countries that*

pertained to the children of Israel, and made all that were
present in Israel to serve, even to serve the Lord their God.
And all his days they departed not from following the Lord,
the God of their fathers." (2 Chron. 34:33)

Though all men have souls, all have not attained to the
position of worshipping the one true God. Many are where
Josiah was before he found the Word of God in the temple.
They have a belief in some higher power, whether it be a nature god or merely their own higher mind. They do what
they think is right in their own sight and it is amazing how
many people, who consider themselves Christians, are actually in this category. There are degrees of "soul stature"
and these are evident by the level of awareness of the individual and by the nature of things to which he is drawn.

The levels of soul awareness are categorized as: *the brutish*
(Psa. 92:6; Prov. 30:2; Jude 10; Jer. 10:21); *the human soul*
(Job 4:17; Cor. 15:47; James 3:15); *the psychical* (examples:
Balaam, a soothsayer, Deut. 23:4; Witch of Endor, 1 Sam.
28:7-25); *the rational soul* (1 Cor. 3:18; Col. 2:8; Matt.
11:25); *the illumined* (examples are apparent in the lives of
Moses, Isaiah, Ezekial, Daniel and John the Revelator) *and*
the Divine which is complete in Jesus Christ.

The lower categories are those of the spiritually unawak-
ened man who has not become aware of God's guidance of
his soul.

"For what man knoweth the things of a man, save the
spirit of man which is in him? Even so the things of God
knoweth no man, but the Spirit of God. Now we have
received, not the spirit of the world, but the spirit which is

of God; that we might know the things that are freely given to us of God. Which things also we speak, not in words which man's wisdom teacheth, but which the Holy Ghost teacheth; comparing spiritual things with spiritual. But the natural man receiveth not the things of the Spirit of God: for they are foolishness unto him: neither can he know them, because they are spiritually discerned. But he that is spiritual judgeth all things, yet he himself is judged of no man." (1 Cor. 2:11-15)

God is Spirit and speaks to us through our spirits. Our spirits can comprehend what God says, but our minds cannot. They cannot even imagine the things which God would speak to our spirits. So our spirits speak to our souls, impressing upon the heart of the soul the glories held for us in heaven, reminding us now one way and then another, that we must not tarry in this search for our identity or we may get lost and delay our journey homeward. *"But there is a spirit in man: and the inspiration of the Almighty giveth them understanding."* (Job 32:8)

But what forces are engaged upon the human and divine co-existing in one body. *"For which cause we faint not; but though our outward man perish, yet the inward man is renewed day by day."* (2 Cor. 4:16) Because the flesh was raised up out of the earth, we are told, it does not recoil at the idea of dust returning to dust. It is the soul of man who rejects the thought of death because it intuitively knows that God had a more perfect plan in mind when He caused the soul to indwell the house of clay.

The account of Joshua (1 Chron. 7:27) reveals God's plan

in the allegory of an historical event. In Hebrew, the names Joshua and Jesua (Jesus) are identical. Both of these names are derived from the word "Jehovah," meaning "I AM THAT I AM." The obvious difference between Joshua and Jesus is the extent of conscious realization of identity with the I AM. Jesus had complete surrender to and identification with the Father God. *"I and my Father are one."* (John 10:30) *" . . . he that hath seen me hath seen the Father; . . . "* (John 14:9)

Joshua was a priest, surrendered and willing but lacking the fullness of power which was given to our Lord Jesus because, as man, he was not totally surrendered. Yet, he was given the divine assignment of assisting Moses (the Law Giver) in bringing the children of Israel (religious thought activity which belongs to the soul in man) into Canaan, the Promised Land.

When we are born again of the Spirit, we have the power from on high bequeathed to us according to the promise of Jesus. Through the power of the indwelling Holy Spirit, we are henceforth able to lay hold of and attain to the redemption of our life forces which includes bringing our bodies into submission to the Spirit so that the regenerative work can begin. This is accomplished only through our cooperation with the Holy Spirit. We must, daily, put our increasing gifts of the Spirit to work in harmony with the Holy Spirit and, in this manner, develop the spiritual consciousness. Even as Joshua had to have the complete obedience of *all* the children of Israel before they were permitted to enter into the land of milk and honey, so we must succeed in bringing all our faculties and forces into subservience to the Mind of Christ.

The more we worship in the spirit, feed upon the Word of God, pray without ceasing, use the gifts of the Spirit which have been given, the more we are merged with our own higher forces and with the forces of God. There is a definitive plan of redemption which is not without our agreement and cooperation. *Whosoever will* may enter into the Plan of God, but no one is forced to do so. Those who are in rebellion to the will of God will not enter into Canaan Land, any more than those disobedient Israelites. The whole enactment of Moses, the children of Israel and Joshua tells us, in an unforgettable manner, that there must first be an obedience to the Law of God, then a purification of the mind of man, accompanied with sacrifices and a total obedience to God, before there can be the regeneration of the body.

Moses represents the Law of God which can take us only so far in the grand work of the soul, for Moses was not permitted to enter into Canaan. Joshua represents that spiritualized consciousness in man which can only come about by the baptism of the Holy Spirit. *"And Joshua the son of Nun was full of the spirit of wisdom; for Moses had laid his hands upon him. . . . "* (Deut. 34:9) Until that time, man may follow the letter of the law, but he is still only man, belonging to this world. Jesus said, *"Except a man be born again, he cannot see the kingdom of God."* (John 3:3)

We see, then, the tremendous burden of responsibility placed upon the soul, for the soil must be prepared to receive the spiritual seed which is sown into the life of mortal man.

That "soil" is the heart, the seat of the *inner man* which acts as a bridge between the mortal awareness and the spirit of man.

The spirit of man knows the purpose of life and the Plan of God. *"The spirit truly is ready, but the flesh is weak."* (Mark 14:38) Also see Luke 22:40. The soul stands in the "great divide" between the world of spirit and the world of flesh, seeing more than the mortal can see, knowing what is ahead if that ego self does not respond to the spiritual call, "Come home, come home. Ye who are weary, come home."

How many times does the call go unanswered? "Almost persuaded . . . now to believe." How many times may one refuse to respond before he becomes hardened?

Our souls are vitally concerned with the way we act and react to circumstances, because the manner in which the ego responds may well effect the future destiny of the soul. Why should the mortal ego be concerned about eternity? The temporal and earthy are given only the short duration of a lifetime to work out its choice of destiny. Then it dissolves and disappears as a vapour. But the life of the soul is designed to be longer than a mere earthly incarnation. There are many mansions, Jesus said, and it is the soul which is destined to stand before the Great White Throne someday.

"For we know that if our earthly house of this tabernacle were dissolved, we have a building of God, a house not made with hands, eternal in the heavens. Therefore we are always confident, knowing that, whilst we are at home in the body, we are absent from the Lord: (For we walk by faith, not by sight:) For we must all appear before the judgment seat of

Christ; that every one may receive the things done in his body, according to that he hath done, whether it be good or bad." (2 Cor. 5:1, 6-7, 10)

In order to put our lives under the directorship of our souls, so that we may be led by the Holy Spirit and through Him come to perfection, we will have to understand the nature of man . . . of self. Contrary to common belief, we are not just "human nature," even though that may be all of the self of which we are aware. Nor does recognizing that we "have souls" open us to the guidance of the *inner man.* Our souls may be working at overcoming far beyond the level of the development of the mortal self. And it is this mortal self, consisting of the ego, personality and intellect, which must be crucified, in order that the spiritual man may be lifted up.

However, without a glimpse of the inner man, consciously or unconsciously, who would ascribe to such a theory? It is an unusual strain of people who, under the spell of religious fervor, would surrender all that they possess of wealth, fame, comfort to pursue some intangible "calling."

Yet, that is exactly what happens. Once that "inner splendor" is perceived or felt, the individual enters into another dimension of life which makes him or her more than mortal. He has been impregnated with the germ of divinity and his offspring shall be the "new creature," the child of God. And the soul of man, clothed in the wedding garment, without spot or wrinkle, becomes the willing bride of Christ.

Not everyone consciously "sees" or feels the activity of the soul, but I believe, without exception, that those who

have experienced God's forgiveness have a new sense of moral
and ethical value, a deepening of the faculty of love, an eleva-
tion of the entire mortal nature, a sense of joy and identification of beauty, and an increase in devotional inclination.
What else could cause a person to change so suddenly?

My own experience was the culmination of several years of
intense spiritual searching. Having lost my first born child,
suddenly and without preparation, I found that the tenets of
my faith did not sustain me. I needed to know, without
reservation, what happened to a person when they died. Did
they continue to live in another world or did they sleep
until the resurrection? Or was there nothing but oblivion?
The three pastors of the church I was attending at that time
could not agree on an answer for me.

I studied the Bible, read countless hundreds of books on
philosophy and theology, studied all the major religions of
the world, prayed, contemplated and meditated, and one
night, the answer came. I became aware of my immortal soul.

I will not go into detail now, concerning this unusual
experience. Suffice it to say, that after a succession of extraordinary events consisting of divine leading, I saw, with
my physical eyes, my illumined soul, and the memory of it
still brings deep longing in me.

At the time of the experience I had full consciousness as
my level of identity shifted from the physical to the soul part
of me. I knew that my soul was the real me, as I was intended
to be — without limitations and the bufferings of the body.
I was in a body which was as completely formed as the
physical body. I had all the faculties of the senses, although

they were much more sensitive and finely tuned. Whatever I sensed through my "soul" was intensified from that which I would have experienced in the flesh.

I could see all around me in all directions at once as if my body were covered with eyes. The depth of love and joy was so great, I thought my heart would burst. I was able to feel, as though they were my own, the emotions of other souls moving upon the etheric waves surrounding me and my heart responded to each emotion. It was as if my heart was a finely tuned harp and all those emotions of my spiritual kin were playing a song of human suffering and delight which I could share with every living creature. I then understood how it was that God could know and be touched by all our cares at once.

I could also feel the impact of every thought which floated by me on the thought waves which surround us all. Each thought, depending upon the content of it, seemed to make a corresponding sound within my being, that of either sadness or joy.

But the most amazing of all that I beheld of my soul was the substance of which the body was made! It was fashioned of light! Pure radiant white light! My head and face were light! My arms and legs and trunk were light! I held out my hands and examined them front and back, marvelling at the iridescence of them. I was in a solid body even though it was luminous and nearly transparent. I knew that this was not the glorified, incorruptible body which we shall have when Jesus comes again and we are translated. This was the body of my soul and it was complete for the plane upon which it was assigned.

I loved the way I felt, being pure soul, with mortality temporarily laid aside, and the hindrance of the heavy flesh taken away. I wanted to stay that way forever, totally merged with my soul, with it having the dominance over the Joyce part of me. But I had to come back and take up the flesh once again.

This one fact has been indelibly imprinted upon every cell of my being: my soul is functioning so far beyond what Joyce is doing. Then, twelve years ago, I didn't know how to get my mortal self up to where my soul is. I had no hope of attaining that because no matter how I tried to do right and sin not, I fell flat on my face every single day in one way or another.

Thanks be to God, after wandering in the wilderness, the Lord led me out, baptized me with the Holy Spirit and has been working to sanctify me. With the Holy Spirit working within me and my heart desiring with all urgency to have the fullness of Christ, I shall one day be a whole and unified being, complete in His Image; body, soul and spirit redeemed!

I have heard some teachers and evangelists of today say, we must not be "soulish" . . . we should be spiritual. But, the spirit of man works through the soul even as mind and feeling operate through the physical body. Have you ever seen a heart or a mind running around by themselves? Neither does our spirit operate on this earthly plane without the soul and the body. These teachers, not understanding what makes up the whole human being, are probably classifying this teaching with the lower categories of soul which seek sensual stimuli. Whatever position is taken, there never will be an occasion when the mortal part of man will be more advanced than his soul.

Yet the majority of mankind stumbles in his darkness. so entangled by the delusion which he believes to be his life, that he cannot grasp the meaning of his immortal soul. *"For the Lord hath poured out upon you the spirit of deep sleep, and hath closed your eyes: the prophets and your rulers, the seers hath he covered. And the vision of all is become unto you as the words of a book that is sealed, which men deliver to one that is learned, saying, 'Read this, I pray thee: and he saith, I cannot; for it is sealed': . . . "* (Isa. 29:10-12) *"They have not known nor understood: for he hath shut their eyes, that they cannot see; and their hearts, that they cannot understand. And none considereth in his heart, neither is there knowledge nor understanding to say, I have burned part of it in the fire; yea, also I have baked bread upon the coals thereof; I have roasted flesh, and eaten it: and shall I make the residue thereof an abomination? Shall I fall down to the stock of a tree? He feedeth on ashes: a deceived heart hath turned him aside, that he cannot deliver his soul, nor say, Is there not a lie in my right hand?"* (Isa. 44:18-20)

There are two objectives for the soul which are assigned by the Creator who gave it Life:

1. To have conscious recognition from the mortal part of self, and

2. To have the freedom of spiritual expression for itself.

Without these two opportunities, the soul is bound and full

of anguish. *"My people are destroyed for lack of knowledge: because thou hast rejected knowledge, I will also reject thee, that thou shalt be no priest to me: . . . therefore the people that doth not understand shall fall."* (Hos. 4:6, 14)

The knowledge which the soul must have for nourishment comes from digesting the Word of God. This is the Bread of Life, the spiritual food which increases the strength of the soul so that it is able to withstand the trials and lessons which the mortal part of self must endure. The Word of God is the only food which the soul can digest and assimilate because it "leadeth to all wisdom." Without the Word, the experiences of life are lost as learning processes to the soul. It can develop no wisdom because there is no foundation of precept to build upon.

Without this nourishment and opportunity for expression, the soul becomes weak and its energy is dissipated. It becomes subjective to the personality of the self who will then choose its own pattern of living with no regard for the future of its immortal self.

Once the personality begins to exercise this kind of dominance over the soul, there will begin a tremendous struggle and the conscience will be overactive in an effort to keep the personality within the bounds of God's law. *"Also, that the soul be without knowledge, it is not good; . . . The foolishness of man perverteth his way: and his heart fretteth against the Lord."* (Prov. 19:2-3)

As the personality wins one round of conflict after another, the soul becomes battle fatigued and weakened and the conscience less active until the mortal self has all but won the dominant role. Some people will then choose the path leading away from God, even though at one time they knew the law of God and were sensitive to the suggestions of the soul. As they walk a road which takes them down hill more and more toward the pull of the earth's vibration, they have all but given up conscience. No longer are they tormented when they willfully break commandments. Their souls are lying sick, near starvation and unable to exert an influence over the mortal self. *"For my people is foolish, they have not known me; they are sottish children, and they have none understanding: they are wise to do evil, but to do good they have no knowledge."* (Jer. 4:22)

Ezekial (12:2), calling the soul "the son of man," addresses the situation: *"Son of man, thou dwellest in the midst of a rebellious house, which have eyes to see, and see not; they have ears to hear, and hear not: for they are a rebellious house."* The house which Ezekial refers to is, of course, the mortal man. Such souls are in danger of death or being over-taken by demonic spirits because they have not enough strength to protect their "houses." They have no moderator to protect them from negative influences. Without response from an awakened soul, God is not able to communicate with man and the mortal self is without guidance and divine influence. There is nothing which will seem wrong to them any longer. Abortion is right, adultery is fun, lying is a matter of course, getting what the personality wants at any cost is the order of the day. Drunkeness becomes a physical ailment requiring sympathy and understanding: homosexuality is a personal choice and blasphemy is just a cute way of talking.

Once a person gains this much control over his immortal soul, he is capable of doing anything. And we have more and more people on this earth today who have fallen into this state. We read of the atrocities they have committed and we shudder, wondering how anyone could do such terrible things. It doesn't happen all at once. It is a gradual falling away. It is a refusal of the influence of the soul when it first activates the conscience and tells the person that what they are doing is wrong. It is turning away from the conviction of the Holy Spirit.

It is following after the mores of the society and allowing the rational mind to be influenced by group opinion, declaring that this activity can't be too bad because everyone is doing it.

All things begin with something small and inconsequential and move by steps and degrees until they become stupendous. So it is with the embracing of evil, and the killing of the immortal soul.

Many people erroneously believe that the intellect and the soul are synonomous. The intellect, however, is what is accumulated by the mortal part of man through his five senses. The intellect judges things from the outward appearance and is, consequently, often deceived. Intuition, an aspect of the soul, corrects the intellect by reminding man that things are not always as they appear to be. *"But the natural man* (or the intellectual man) *receiveth not the things of the Spirit of God: for they are foolishness unto him: neither can he know them, because they are spiritually discerned."* (1 Cor. 2:14)

Intellectual understanding is not wrong. We need a developed mind in order to live a fruitful life in this physical world; the mistake we often make is putting all our trust in the intellect for the reason that it does deal only with the physical world. We are spiritual beings who have souls. Our realm of origin is spirit and spirit *cognizes.* Our realm of expression is soul and soul *intuits.* Our realm of manifestation is physical and the physical *reasons.* *"Trust in the Lord with all thine heart* (soul), *and lean not unto thine own understanding."* (Prov. 3:5)

We come to understand, therefore, that what we know at the personality level has gone through several processes before we embraced it as an idea of our own. All knowledge does not come from books or from the minds of great teachers. The only knowledge which will abide with us at the intellectual level is that which has been received both spiritually and emotionally. That which is learned merely by rote is meaningless. It has no quickening power. It cannot change our lives or the lives of others. That is why, today, there are so many powerless religious leaders. They may have gone through seminary, attained degrees, have the command of memory to be able to quote from books and speakers; but they may never win a soul to Christ. It is only the spiritually quickened Word of God which can convert a man at the level of his soul. *"For the word of God is quick, and powerful, and sharper than any two-edged sword, piercing even to the dividing asunder of soul and spirit, and of the joints and marrow, and is a discerner of the thoughts and intents of the heart."* (Heb. 4:12)

The intellect of man must be redeemed from its identification with sense perception in order to bring about His "kingdom on earth as it is in heaven." This begins with an intellectual baptism . . . a washing with the water of the Word. We consciously pray to rid ourselves of the negative thought patterns which have been established in us and have been responsible for much of the misery we have known. Then, the mind is renewed with positive decrees of righteousness and virtue (whatsoever things are true, etc.), until we are transformed.

The intellectual part of man is influenced by the soul when he permits it to be. He finds that he gathers data by a process which is often automatic and subliminal. He gets a "hunch" which defies what he knows, intellectually, and makes a decision based upon it and finds it to be correct. Few people are aware, however, that these "hunches" are the intuitive impressions of the soul, guiding the personality to its ultimate good.

The soul has its own language for communicating, an ancient language which is the basis for all communication: symbology. Symbols are pictures which represent whole concepts to the soul. These symbol pictures may be transmitted to us, so proficiently, that we are not even aware that we are seeing them, yet they make their impression upon the mind and we are influenced by them.

For this reason, the Bible presents symbols to us. Although all the stories and people are real and their experiences are historically true, each person and the unique part they played in the epic of the spiritual development of the children of

God is, at the same time, a symbolic presentation to us for our spiritual direction. The Bible is intimately personal. That is why it alone has the power to deliver us from the bondage which our souls have endured. Like the Israelites who were in bondage in Egypt, we are being set free, but our freedom comes individually, as we awaken to who we are in the Lord.

Because Moses stood on the mountaintop and saw the Promised Land, we, too, have stood there. We have seen grapes from the brook, Eschcol, and have heard the good report that it is, indeed, a land of milk and honey. And the best part of the report is that Canaan is not in heaven. Canaan is here on earth! Even though that land is peopled with the negative forces of the carnal world (the Hittites, the Hivites, the Jebusites and the Amorites), the Word says, *"Let us go up at once, and possess it; for we are well able to overcome it. . . ."* (Nu. 13:30)

Don't listen to the evil report of the giants in the land. We have a mighty calling to be the giants in the land and *"If the Lord delight in us, then he will bring us into this land, and give it to us; a land which floweth with milk and honey. Only rebel not ye against the Lord, neither fear ye the people of the land; for they are bread for us: their defence is departed from them, and the Lord is with us: fear them not."* (Nu. 14:8-9)

Several months ago, the Spirit of the Lord spoke to my heart saying these words, "BEHOLD! I AM RAISING UP A MIGHTY ARMY TO DO BATTLE FOR ME, AND YE SHALL BE FITTED WITH AN ARMOUR FOR WAR.

WEAPONS YE SHALL HAVE OF SPIRIT AND OF FIRE
TO DO BATTLE FOR ME, IN THESE LATTER DAYS,
AS YE ARE CALLED TO OVERCOME THE CHILDREN
OF DARKNESS. I HAVE DELIVERED THEM INTO YOUR
HANDS, AND I COMMAND, GO! AND TAKE YE THE
LAND!"

The children of God have been warriors on this earth.
They have not stood back and permitted Satan's army to
possess the land. Armed in righteousness, the children of
God have never doubted that when God said, *"The earth is
the Lord's, and the fullness thereof; . . . "* (Psa. 24:1) He
meant it for us, His chosen people. Then why should we
delay any longer in claiming this blood-washed land?

Now the Law Giver says if you would receive your inheritance in the land of Canaan, you must first go over
Jordan, the River of Judgment, according to the Hebrew.
You cannot possess the land without crossing the river. The
Lord is telling us that the Land of Promise is awaiting us but,
before we can lay claim to that ancient inheritance, we must
permit ourselves to objectively judge ourselves – consciously
and subconscioulsy. We must figuratively, walk through the
River Jordan and be washed clean. In an earlier chapter, we
covered the truth that before one can be converted, there
must first be a realization of sin, confession and repentance.

If we do not believe that we have sinned we would have
nothing to confess. That is where the judgment of self comes
into play. For forty years, as he tended the sheep in Midian,
Moses went through the process of self-judgement. When he
had completed this introspection, he came to the foot of the

Mount Horeb.

Until we judge ourselves, we are in a spiritually dry place —
a desert. As we come face to face with the righteousness of
God, through His Word, we see how unrighteous we are. The
truth of His Word reveals us to ourselves and we are judged
by the judicial faculty of our own intelligence. And when we
see ourselves as we truly are, we are ready to step into the
Jordan, "the descending river from above," which is a type of
the Rivers of Living Waters of which Jesus spoke.

Empowered by the Holy Spirit, the flowing of judgment
no longer holds a fear for us. For we know that we are redeemed by His blood, even before we realized it. When we
know this at all levels of consciousness, we are able to cross
over to the other side.

*"And ye shall dispossess the inhabitants of the land, and
dwell therein: for I have given you the land to possess it.
But if ye will not drive out the inhabitants of the land from
before you; then it shall come to pass, that those which ye
let remain of them shall be pricks in your eyes, and thorns
in your sides, and shall vex you in the land wherein ye dwell.
Moreover it shall come to pass, that I shall do unto you,
as I thought to do unto them."* (Nu. 33:53, 55-56)

The children of God look to two cities as places of blessing
and sanctuary: Canaan and Jerusalem. The New Jerusalem
descending from the clouds, pristine and pure, full of glory,
excites the believer. My spirit leaps up in joy at the mention
of it. Jerusalem is a spiritual retreat, a four-dimensional
creation made for us when we become four-dimensional
beings in glorified bodies. It is also symbolic of the spirit of

man in its full glory when it is wedded to Christ.

But Canaan is three-dimensional. Canaan is physical. It is a retreat for us while we are yet in the physical body and this physical, three-dimensional world. It is waiting for us to claim it. But we do not claim it by just resting on spiritual promises. To the contrary, God is revealing to us that Jerusalem cannot be a reality until we have possessed Canaan.

To possess Canaan, which is symbolic of the redeemed soul which is expressing the fruits of the Spirit, we must overcome the limitations of the physical world. We must "drive out" the enemy forces inhabiting this "land," those which hold the soul in retreat and from claiming that which God has ordained. Those enemy forces are negativism, the belief in duality, the yielding to the power of Satan through sickness, sin and death. Only then will we be able to bring about the good intentions planted within our spirits so that we can be transformed into imperishable, incorruptible beings.

All that we have studied in the early account of the patriarchs indicates that man has been placed in this physical world to learn and to grow, to overcome and to submit completely to the Will of God. And, in so doing, he will enter into a covenant with God which will bring about everlasting life. Isn't it about time we all went down to the River Jordan?

9

The Choice Is Yours.

Forty years Moses was in the backside of the desert. This man of genteel breeding and sun-protected skin wore the forelock of a prince of Egypt. His work was tending sheep in the desert of Midian, and, as he moved about doing his chores he grew in strength and stature until he was prepared for the calling he had received from God.

No one chooses to go to a desert. It is a hot and dry and lonely place. It is a place where there is little water to quench one's thirst. But desert experiences come to all of us. When we are in a desert experience we discover that it doesn't have to be a dry place after all. Deserts can bloom like a rose.

A desert's vista is monotonous in its barrenness. With nothing to beguile our attention outwardly, we are forced to look inward. When we do, we begin to discover ourselves.

In our culture, very little is said of self-awareness. The term seldom comes up, even in our most devout religious

training. We are taught religious practices which involve the
mind, the body and the senses but these are merely disciplines. And disciplines cannot acquaint us with who we really
are or who God is.

Moses was raised as a prince of Egypt, taskmaster of the
Hebrews, but the clothes and jewelry did not make him an
Egyptian. His blood was the blood of a Jew. And when he
realized the truth of his blood line he left the land of his
birth for the backside of a desert.

We are not what we appear to be on the surface, either.
Nor are we what we think ourselves to be. The Jewish blood
which flowed through the veins of Moses is symbolical of
the spirit which flows through us which determines our true
identity. When we awaken to the truth that we are not the
flesh we think ourselves to be, but rather spirit, we consciously move out of the world of matter into the realm of
spirit. But we find that it is necessary to spend some time
in the sanctuary of the desert.

It is not easy to be in the desert. It is a time when we feel
all is lost and we are left alone with nothing but our thoughts
and the memories stored in the subconscious. Yet it is this
very condition which causes us to establish the great and
lasting truth of our true identity which we would never have
found if we had not gone into the desert.

The physical body, with its limited time for life and
expression, wants to hold onto every moment – to live
to the fullest and experience that which pleases the flesh.
Eat more, drink more, smoke more, frolic more. "Sub-
merge in a sea of pleasure," the body says, "for tomor-

row we may die." This is the land of Egypt. The world of materialism and carnality. But a child of God cannot stay in that world. He would rather sit alone in the desert. And he chooses the desert . . . or perhaps the desert chooses him . . . because the soul within knows its true identity and the home from which it has departed and longs to return to its native land.

The belief that life is experienced only through the body and its senses is the great Satanic lie which has bound humanity since Eden. It is a delusion — one which has been so perpetrated upon human life that few can conceive the truth of being and allow the real self to step forth and claim the life ordained for him through the victory of Jesus Christ.

We say with our mouths that we believe that we are spirit having souls which live in physical bodies, but we fail to grasp the very essence of this truth so that we can live as though we believe. We catch wispy glimpses of the truth and, almost immediately, some bodily urge pulls us back to the dominance of the flesh.

There are theosophical movements which deny the existence of the body. In fact, they deny the existence of anything which is comprised of matter. To them, matter is evil and spirit is good so they deny the power of matter by denying its existence.

But God created matter. And, in our Christian teaching, we find a marvelous mysterious revelation which has not been revealed to any other mystical or philosophical movement. Paul alludes to this revelation when he says, *"Behold, I show you a mystery; We shall not all sleep, but we shall all*

be changed, In a moment, in the twinkling of any eye, at the
last trump: . . . " (1 Cor. 15:51) *"For this corruptible must*
put on incorruption, and this mortal must put on immortal-
ity. So when this corruptible shall have put on incorruption,
and this mortal shall have put on immortality, then shall be
brought to pass the saying that is written, Death is swallowed
up in victory." (1 Cor. 15:53-54)

It is possible to break the bondage of the flesh. The very
first step in doing so is . . . "SEEK GOD!"

Jesus said the kingdom of God is within. If we are to
seek God, it is only sensible that we begin to look for Him
where He may be found . . . within . . . as Jesus said. And as
we look within, one by one we begin to break the chains of
bondage to sense awareness. Within, we discover the REAL
SELF, the vehicle God gave to our individualized spirits by
which we were able to become self-aware.

Even though Moses was raised as a prince of Egypt, he
was nurtured and taught by his real mother, an Israelite of
the Levite tribe. We know that she privately taught him all
the stories of the God of Israel and the patriarchs. As his
natural mother, she must have found it difficult not to
reveal their elite heritage. But Moses didn't identify with
the Israelites until he was forty years old. He spent all that
time being an Egyptian. And he became converted when he
faced who he really was. No longer was he an Egyptian. He
was a child of God!

We can belong to a church, go there every Sunday, read
the Bible daily and still not be a child of God. We have to
have an experience of conversion, NEW BIRTH IN CHRIST,

before we are ready and willing to leave Egypt land . . . the land of materiality and carnality, and take on our true identity.

Becoming converted means changing our focal center from the physical to the soul, the inner man. Basically, this is what happens at conversion. We may have been religious, but it was a mere discipline of mind and body. Good disciplines naturally ensure us good attitudes which bring a measure of good health and a robust body. Many worldly people enjoy excellent health because of the disciplines they apply.

Physical disciplines are good for us but they don't make us spiritual or aware of spiritual matters. They help keep us at the level of the physical, which is how we tend to look at the world . . . from our own focal point, at the level of the flesh and ego. This makes us self-centered. Everything we experience is measured by our point of view, our own understanding, our own concepts, prejudices, beliefs. Some of them may be right; some of them may be completely wrong. But, in the natural, we are unaware of our error. WE are the center of our universe.

When we are converted, we begin to see things differently. We are given a new mind and a new heart which is in Christ Jesus. Our focal point is now transferred to the soul. The soul of man knows that God is the center of the universe and everything must be measured against Him.

This is when we see one's life change. Who among us can stand in the Presence of Almighty God and still consider himself to be anything in his own merit? Who among us can hold onto his self-made ideas of nothingness when his soul has

become cognizant of the radiant and majestic holy creation
of our Creator's unutterable glory. And who, upon perceiving
a glimpse of this glory, however dim it may be as seen
through the clouds of our long delusion, can continue to
count his own awkward creation of anything valuable enough
to sustain?

The soul who has heard even a whisper of angels' voices no
longer desires to place complete dependency upon this world
of form and matter. That soul yearns to surrender all the
worthlessness it previously called "self" to become lost in
the endless, boundless, bottomless love of our precious
Father God.

This is not to say that we should ascribe to a teaching of
self-abnegation. To the contrary; such a practice of symbolically or literally flailing oneself to bring "the wicked
flesh" into submission can and usually does develop psychic
aberrations which can damage the mind as well as the body.
If we follow the Pauline teachings, upon which all Christian
theology is based, we can see the advocation of redemption
rather than the denial of the senses and the flesh.

Paul said, *"Not as though I had already attained, either
were already perfect: but I follow after, if that I may ap-
prehend that for which also I am apprehended of Christ
Jesus. Brethren, I count not myself to have apprehended:
but this one thing I do, forgetting those things which are
behind, and reaching forth unto those things which are
before, I press toward the mark for the prize of the high
calling of God in Christ Jesus. Let us therefore, as many
as be perfect, be thus minded: and if in any thing ye be*

otherwise minded, God shall reveal even this unto you.
(Phil. 3:12-15)

What encouragement! We haven't reached the goal yet, but we hold fast to the belief that, if we are called to this divine purpose of perfection in Christ, it shall be done! We don't have to look back at the mistakes we may have made, nor do we think of the life we lived "in the world." That is over and done with. Looking back serves only to "turn us into a pillar of salt." And should we, even momentarily, look back to "the world"? *"Did ever people hear the voice of God speaking out of the midst of the fire, as thou hast heard, and live?"* (Deut. 4:33) The children of Almighty God are blessed indeed. We have the Comforter to personally guide us through life so that we don't fall out of grace.

Moses was called from out of the desert to go back to Egypt and lead the Israelites out of that land. He was to lead them to the land of Canaan which had been promised to them through Abraham. That land wasn't sitting there fallow and unoccupied, waiting for them to be released from Egyptian captivity. There were strongholds of great tribes and nations. Archeological discoveries of recent years reveal the ruins of hundreds of fortified cities which covered the hills of Moab, Ammon and Gilead.

Yet, God told the Children of Israel to go in and possess the land. *"To drive out nations from before thee greater and mightier than thou art, to bring thee in, to give thee their land for an inheritance, as it is this day."* (Deut. 4:38) In order to possess the land, the Israelites had to cast out the Hittites, the Girgashites, the Amorites, the Canaanites, the

Perizzites, the Hivites, and the Jebusites.

The Hittites represent terror, the Girgashites represent materialism; ethnocentricity is the idea represented by the Amorites who boasted being descended from Noah; Perizzites are symbolical of sense consciousness, the Hivites stand for bestiality or wickedness and the Jebusites are representative of the state of subjection or profanity.

It is our responsibility to drive out from our "land" . . . the mortal mind and consequently the body . . . those states of consciousness and emotional attitudes which relate to the world of darkness and sense attachment. We must see that it is done. No one else can do it for us. Our minds are our responsibility and it is for us to establish God's kingdom in our mind. *"Ye shall observe to do therefore as the Lord your God hath commanded you: ye shall not turn aside to the right hand or to the left. Ye shall walk in all the ways which the Lord your God hath commanded you, that ye may live, and that it may be well with you, and that ye may prolong your days in the land which ye shall possess.* (Deut. 5:32-33)

It should have taken only eleven days for the Israelites to journey from Egypt to Canaan. Instead, with the Promised Land right within reach, they wandered in the wilderness for forty more years and Moses died, "his eye was not dim, nor his natural force abated." He died without ever setting foot in Canaan.

Our Promised Land lies just that close. We wander in the wilderness because we have not overcome all the trials and tribulations confronting us. We have not spent enough time in the desert evaluating ourselves to discover who we are, what we are, and why we meet life the way we do. We have avoided facing the truth of ourselves. We have continually bowed down before idols of golden calves or bronze serpents, even though the law has been presented to us upon the tablets of stone within our hearts, even though the Lord has spoken in the midst of us and we can see the fire and hear the thunder of His glory atop the mountain.

The golden calf is a representative of materialism. This can include, not only our attachment to the material wealth of this world, our material possessions, but in a deeper sense, it represents our attachment to life in the physical and the deeply ingrained belief that without the body there is no life.

Moses had to go up to the top of the mountain to receive the law of God. He had to ascend, in order to meet the Creator and speak to Him face to face.

Frequently, people question why their prayers are not answered. They kneel publicly, cry aloud, speak in tongues but nothing is availed. They are like the children of Israel, dancing around a golden calf at the foot of the mountain. Their prayers have not gone beyond the mortal part of themselves. They haven't met Him in the Spirit.

Several weeks ago, while preparing some soup, the lid blew off my pressure cooker while I was carrying it from the stove to the sink. The steaming liquid went everywhere in the kitchen, scalding my left arm and hand, my right hand, my right leg and both feet. Three fingers on my left hand were singed white.

I attempted to clean up this horrible mess before taking care of my burns. That involved mopping gallons of soup up from the floor, and washing the cupboards, walls, ceiling, and all the appliances. It took over an hour and a half. All the while that I was working, I was affirming God's divine order in the universe. I was in excruciating pain, as you can well imagine. Scaldings are particularly painful and every time I put my hands in the scrub water, the burns intensified. Finally, I could stand the pain no longer.

I sat down and prayed, "Dear Lord, I need your help at once. I am in terrible pain. I know that you hear me and that it is not your desire for me to suffer. Therefore, in the name of Jesus Christ I ask for complete healing, at once, according to the Words spoken to us by your Son. And now, that I may glorify Jesus on this earth, even as He glorifies you in Heaven I await complete healing and give you all the honor, praise and glory, in Jesus Name. Amen."

Then, I went in the Spirit "up to the mountaintop," where I met my God and my Healer. I stayed there for about five minutes and when I came down, the pain was completely gone, there was not a blister, red mark or soreness as evidence of the scalding! I was completely healed! It was finished in that moment and nothing more needed to be done except to praise God who hears and answers our prayers. I was able to get up immediately and, without further discomfort, I resumed my cleaning. I have glorified my God again and again as I testified to many people concerning this miraculous healing.

My prayers, for the hour and a half while I was cleaning up the mess in my kitchen, were not enough. I had to meet the Lord on the mountaintop. That meant going into my "prayer closet" deep within where the transcendent glory of God abides in the sanctuary of my spiritual heart. *"Now the Lord is the Spirit: and where the Spirit of the Lord is, there is liberty."* (2 Cor. 3:17) *"For it is God who said, 'Let light shine out of darkness,' who has shone in our hearts to give the light of the knowledge of the glory of God in the face of Christ. But we have this treasure in earthen vessels, to show that the transcendent power belongs to God and not to us."* (2 Cor. 4:6-7 R.S.V.)

Although most Christians do not know how to go within and ask that the transcendent power of God heal them, the time is come when we will respond, in greater numbers, to receive His grace and to *". . . worship the Father in spirit and truth: for the Father seeketh such to worship him."* (John 4:23)

The prayers which proceed out of our mouths and emotions are equivalent to the children of Israel dancing around a golden calf at the foot of the mountain, and, frequently, this is the reason we don't get results.

While Moses was on the mountaintop, talking with God, the people became restless. They didn't know to whom to turn for help in their spiritual life, and because Aaron couldn't go up the mountain, he answered their needs with a golden calf.

"Going up on the mountaintop" means rising above the cares of this world, above our negative, worrisome thought processes, above our response to pain and above our attachment to physical, material things. Aaron either didn't know how to do that himself or didn't know how to lead the people or decided "they weren't ready for that." So he came up with a material, physical substitute.

Isn't this exactly what the pharasaical church has done for so many years? They either didn't know how to go where Moses went, or they knew but decided the people couldn't handle it, so they made golden calves to satisfy their spiritual longing and they've never gotten beyond the foot of the mountain.

As priest, Aaron represents our spiritualized intellect. But, no matter how saturated our intellect becomes with prayers and Scriptures and positive decrees, it is still our natural mind working and that cannot take the place of worshipping God in Spirit and in truth.

Our outward religious practices will not be a substitute for communing with God on a personal basis — "face to face." *"But we all, with open face beholding as in a glass the glory of the Lord, are changed into the same image from glory to glory, even as by the Spirit of the Lord."* (2 Cor. 3:18)

Those who have fashioned the golden calves of today, with rituals, beads, printed prayers, or formalized programs, are quick to denounce those who speak of "religious experience." They beat their chests in frenzy, while screaming that to know God is a matter of faith, not feeling." They speak this way because they have not experienced God in a personal manner. He is someone they know a great deal about, but don't know.

We can make a golden calf of our intellect, fashioning it with priceless jewels of accumulated knowledge and the ability to discourse with great profundity and, even though we give it earnest homage . . . this wealth of religious knowledge . . . it is no more than a golden calf . . . that is, unless we have journeyed up the mountain and met God face to face!

I believe the brazen serpent represents sense consciousness. This, along with the belief in materiality, constitutes the prison of matter which has bound man since time immemorial. It is the second motion of mind away from the perfection and immortality of God. The first, if you remember, was a belief in duality. When man first turned his finite mind away from God, to consider other forces, his initial reaction was fear and shame. With fear there entered into the consciousness of man every other negativity of which the world now abounds. Fearing loss of self, due to his disobedience, man attached himself to the first thing he could find which offered solidarity. His body. And, along with his body, came the sense awareness that that body still had life.

Now, eons later, the false concepts of duality and materiality have so become a part of the consciousness of mankind that only those who have ventured away from the multitudes to scale the mountain alone have the illumination of consciousness to KNOW this undeniable and irrefutable unending truth, "I LIVE AND HAVE MY BEING IN HE WHO HAS MADE ME!"

While wandering in the wilderness the Israelites suffered from the bites of fiery serpents. This intimates that Moses was beginning to have problems with "sin in the camp." Moses was told by God, to fashion a *"fiery serpent, and set it upon a pole: and it shall come to pass, that every one*

that is bitten, when he looketh upon it, shall live . . . "
(Nu. 21:8) We don't have to surrender our will to the desires
of the body. We are to have dominion over the body. Indeed,
we must take control over the flesh and put it under subjection to the will of God.

Moses prayed for the people who had been bitten by the
fiery serpents. They *confessed* their sins and *repented.* Again,
in order for a change to take place, this procedure of confession and repentance is necessary. One blanket confession
doesn't cover all the unrighteousness we will discover about
ourselves as we progress along the spiritual path. Each new
awareness we gain of ourselves and our enslavement to that
which did not originate in God requires a period of confession and repentance. Once we turn our attention within, to
objectively consider self in relation to God and to direct
our love nature toward Christ, who has prepared a way for us
that we might draw nigh unto the Father, a process sets in
which brings us into harmony with the nature of God.

We begin to *feel* the reality of the Father's love for us. It
is no longer a mere intellectual concept. Once experienced,
this divine life force, which is the Almighty Father, literally
floods the inner man and transmutes us, cleanses us, purifies
us and perfects us. The work is done by the Father, but we
must meet Him there on the mountain through our devotion, prayer and meditation. *"As Moses lifted up the serpent
in the wilderness, even so must the Son of man (Christ in
us) be lifted up: . . . "* (John 3:14)

It was nearly twenty years ago that I was taught of the
Spirit of God how to "go upon the mountaintop." It was

after I lost my little six year old son and the Word of God became the greatest strength I had to endure this tragedy. I prayed, poured through Scriptures and asked God for answers to the mysteries of life.

And, as the Scripture was revealed to me, my soul stirred within me and I wanted to know more of the Father. After everyone else was in bed at night, I would sit for an hour of prayer and contemplation. I like to call it "resting in the spirit." I would read a Scripture, seeking a deeper meaning of it and committing it to memory. Then I would close my eyes and meditate upon that Scripture. Night after night, I would do this. Years before I had told the Lord, "Where You lead me, I will follow. I'll go with You all the way," and I meant to keep my word. How long did I put myself under His instruction before I was ready to follow Him all the way? Was it two years, three or perhaps four? No, it was seven years. Seven years of desiring to follow Him, and yet, having so much to lay at the altar of sacrifice.

I knew the Lord was leading me into "Canaan land" (deeper experience) but I had heard the bad report, that there were giants in the land which would make me look as small as a grasshopper. You have heard these reports, too, for Canaan is the realm of the spirit and we have heard that Satan and his fallen angels dwell in this land. We know that Satan was an angel who fell from heavenly realm, and we know that he doesn't dwell in the physical realm, so he must reside in between – in the realm of the spirit. But he didn't create this realm, he only profaned it. *Only rebel not ye against the Lord, neither fear ye the people of the land; for*

*they are bread for us: their defence is departed from them,
and the Lord is with us: fear them not."* (Nu. 14:9) *"And ye
shall dispossess the inhabitants of the land, and dwell therein:
for I have given you the land to possess it."* (Nu. 33:53)

Christians have shied away from discovering the promised
land within. They have allowed the children of darkness; the
Moabites, the Hivites, Hittites, Jebusites and the Canaanites
take over the land, and they have been too weak and scared
to go in and possess the land. Until we "drive out" every
vestige of pagan, idolatrous influences within our "inner
man," it is impossible for us to establish the promised land
within — *a land where we walk in divine health.* God has
given us the promise of health, happiness and prosperity, but
we haven't gone in to possess that land.

We can worship God in Spirit and in truth. But, if we want
to change circumstances in our physical life we have to bring
that Spiritual Power down to the physical level, to let the
Holy Spirit move through us. The spirit works through the
soul and the soul works through the body. If the children
of God do not know how to work with that precious com-
modity of the spiritual realm, creative energy, then they
must settle for the inferior staples given to those who function only at the physical/emotional level.

We can never accomplish "the fullness of the image of
Christ" without turning ourselves completely over to Him.
This does not mean laying only the body or the intellect on
the altar of sacrifice. This is a requirement for the entirety of
our being . . . all that we are. And we shall never be able to
do that as long as we whimper around the golden calf trying

to maintain our sense attachment and materiality.

Even though he served God faithfully and humbly for eighty years, Moses was refused entry into the Promised Land. He sacrificed his inheritance as a prince of Egypt, he carried the tremendous burden of an undedicated people and misinformed staff, he suffered the physical discomforts pertaining to sojourning in the wilderness and still he was refused entry into Canaan. Why?

Moses and the children of Israel journeyed from the wilderness of sin to Rephidim. Rephidim means "place of rest." Too often we get the idea that because we have journeyed "out of sin" that we have no need to go further. We camp at Rephidim, to take a rest. It is here that the enemy can attack us and overcome us because we have made only a temporary encampment. We are not expected to stay at Rephidim. The Amalaks represent the carnal nature in each of us which is always ready to overpower us. And because we have not journeyed far enough to build a permanent fortress in the Lord (Promised Land), we are constantly in danger of succumbing to the carnal desires of the flesh. *"And the Lord said unto Moses, 'Write this for a memorial in a book, and rehearse it in the ears of Joshua: for I will utterly put out the remembrance of Amalek from under heaven.' "* (Ex. 17:14)

There was no water in Rephidim, meaning, in this case, that there was no power. There never is. There is neither power for healing nor providing sustenance for life's energies. And people don't comprehend this. They complain, "I became a Christian. I gave up smoking. I don't go to bars anymore. I go to church every Sunday and prayer meeting on Wednesday. So how is it that I still get sick? Why am I not prosperous? Why isn't my life any better than it was before I became a Christian? IS GOD WITH ME OR NOT?

Some preachers stand up tall and declare, "When you become a Christian, Satan tries to destroy you. Consider your trials a sign that the Lord is going to bless you r-e-a-l good or the devil wouldn't be so scared!"

But, the answer is, you stopped at Rephidim, the resting place. You haven't started to build your permanent fortress in Him. And, until you do, you will wonder as the Israelites did, "IS GOD AMONG US OR NOT?"

Rephidim is a resting place, but it is still a wilderness. Far out in the wilderness where you don't know if God is real or not. You have to come up the mountain to see Him. Moses had been to the mountaintop. He had talked to God face to face. He knew, not in the substance of things hoped for as yet unseen, in reality that God is THE ALL-HOLY ONE OF ISRAEL, and as such, deserves reverence, adoration, and total obedience. Moses, because of the murmuring of the people, slipped back to the level of his carnal self, lost patience, and forgot to lift up the name of God before the people when he struck the rock with the rod. He allowed those unretrievable words to escape his lips.

But Moses learned a lesson in Rephidim. It was a costly lesson, but he wrote it down for our preservation so that we need not make the same mistake. He named the place Massah and Meribah; temptation and strife, so that all future generations would realize that, when we allow ourselves to drift

away from "being in the Spirit as He is in the Spirit" we are
going to fall into temptation and strife, and thereby endanger
the progress of our souls.

It is then that we are forbidden entry into "the inner sanctuary" . . . represented by Kadesh. The carnal man . . . will use
every trick and alibi to keep us out. Without that pilgrimage
to the inner sanctuary, how will we ever be filled again and
gain power to continue to the Promised Land?

It is vitally important to learn how to retreat to Kadesh.
What good is our "spirituality" if it is only working for us
when we are in the congregation of the Lord? What happens
when we are working among the Moabites, the Hittites,
Hivites and Jebusites? Do we allow the Amaleks to overpower us while we sit and whine, "Is God with us or not?"

Kadesh means clean; pure; bright; holy; sacred; sanctified;
consecrated; a place of sanctuary. It is a state of perfection.
It is not the Promised Land. It is not the New Jersusalem.
It is on the way to Canaan. If we never stop at Kadesh to
be spiritually refreshed, we will never be able to enter the
Promised Land. It is here in this pure state of consciousness
which is attainable to each of us that we are able to overcome
the hold the carnal self has upon the consciousness. It is here
also . . . this place of judgement (another name for Kadesh)
that we put off the "old man" and begin to put on Christ.

In Kadesh, this inner sanctuary of pure holiness, we cog-
nize at the deepest level of our being that we as individuals
do nothing, know nothing and are nothing except it be by
the Spirit of God which flows through us by grace and in
which we are immersed. All Christians confess this intel-

lectually, but they do not *know* it, because they have never been to the sanctuary in Kadesh. And the power from on high *cannot* be given unto any of us. New wine cannot be put into old bottles. We must first be made fitting vessels of honor in the house of the Lord.

When you pray for someone and lay hands on him what good does it do if you are speaking from your natural self? The power must come from on High. You have to first enter into the Spirit. There you can see the power. You can call it into you. You can feel your spirit body being filled with the power. Your spiritual heart center expands with the love of Christ (because all things must be done in love.) The light of Christ becomes so bright all around you that this world seems to disappear. You can see the spirit of the one for whom you are praying. You can see what his problem is, the reason for it, whether it is the fullness of time when this can be eliminated, how much power to apply and where to apply it. And the receiver of this power will feel it filling him. Either he will be healed or he will be strengthened to endure or he will be enlightened so that he knows the reason for the affliction and can begin working to align his mind and emotions with the mind of God. And the one who has been used as such an instrument will acknowledge the Holy Spirit as the giver of that power. *You are no more than a vessel.*

Now, there are other folks . . . well meaning, but lacking wisdom and speaking without knowledge . . . who say, when they take up the rod to strike the rock, "Not I, but God in me doest all things." But there is that part of them which is still under the power of the Amalek, saying, "Hey you guys!

Did you see what I just did?"

How many new leaders and teachers have been like Moses? They move in the Spirit of the annointing of God until they get to the place where they are asked to provide water. When they hit the rock and the water comes forth, they just can't help feeling *they* did it. The Holy Spirit has "given them power," to lay hands on the sick and heal them, to annoint them and have them "rest in the Spirit," to pray and have those prayers answered. Many times God withdraws the annointing (the stripping of Aaron of his priestly robes) because the vanity of man becomes inflated. This is a pitfall we must avoid as we journey to the land of Canaan. *"Watch and pray, that ye enter not into temptation: the spirit indeed is willing, but the flesh is weak."* (Matt. 26:41)

And then it's back to the desert. Back to the well in Midian. Back to watch over the "flock" of mortal thoughts, to battle all the tribes surrounding Canaan, to tarry a little longer at the foot of the mountain, to tear out all the tangles of negativity, materiality, sense-consciousness and duality which hides the beautiful sanctuary in the midst of Kadesh. And when you do, you will have that inner cognizance that Living Water is always available to you when your life is established in Him — even when you are stranded in the desert.

10

Open The Door To Your Health.

"And a highway shall be there, and a way, and it shall be called The way of holiness; the unclean shall not pass over it; but it shall be for those: the wayfaring men, though fools, shall not err therein. No lion shall be there, nor any ravenous beast shall go up thereon, it shall not be found there; but the redeemed shall walk there: And the ransomed of the Lord shall return, and come to Zion with songs and everlasting joy upon their heads: they shall obtain joy and gladness and sorrow and sighing shall flee away." (Isa. 35:8-10)

Jesus said the kingdom of God is within. He said that when we pray we should go into a closet. Kadesh, in the midst of the Midianite desert, represents the kingdom of God within which we can experience while we are yet in the body.

Canaan is a land of milk and honey, a place of physical perfection and comfort. Canaan is available to the believer who overcomes the limitations of the mortal self, with its sense awareness, and learns to live and operate out of the inner man. It is a physical place for physical people. Canaan

is situated in the midst of the idol worshippers and the ungodly. The physical people, in Canaan, are the born-again
believers who are walking in His Spirit.

Zion, often used figuratively to identify the Holy City,
is a habitation of peace. There is only one way to Jerusalem,
the city of peace, and that is through Christ. When we have
brought all that we are physically, emotionally, intellectually,
and spiritually, under the dominion of Christ, we have established the I AM THAT I AM consciousness within ourselves.
The personality (Jesus) with its intellect (Golgotha) must be
crucified, before the likeness of Christ is able to be manifested in us.

You, who are sincerely seeking to serve God and bring
forth your share of the harvest, mark this well, lest you be
deceived by teachings seeking ascendancy. These teachers
would have you believe that you have already been given all
that is necessary to put on the fullness of Christ. I heard a
young minister say he had the mind of Christ because the
Word says so. Does it?

Paul said, *"Let every soul be subject unto the higher
powers. For there is no power but of God: the powers that
be are ordained of God. Whosoever therefore resisteth the
power, resisteth the ordinance of God: and they that resist
shall receive to themselves damnation."* (Rom. 13:1-2)

Even the best of us, where we are in our present state of
development, are doing no more than making a yearly
pilgrimage to Jerusalem to visit the temple. Sometimes we
stand in the outer court, which is reserved for the Gentiles.
Sometimes we stand up to teach, but we are doing no more

than periodically bringing about a spiritualized condition in the physical temple of stone and mortar.

Moses was a type of all mankind and man's journey back to God. Solomon was a type of Jesus. He built "the house of the Lord and his own house" in Jerusalem. He signified what man, operating at the spiritual level of consciousness, could do when he is surrendered to the will of God. Solomon typifies man at a higher level of spiritual development than what Moses was.

Jesus completes the scenario which was begun at the dawn of creation and carries the plan of God through to divine fulfillment. Not only has He bought back the souls of all mankind from the power of the enemy, He has shown the way whereby we may have perfect peace in Him.

The Holy Temple in Jerusalem represents the center of love in the consciousness of man. Without love, man is not able to progress beyond the level of brute. Love is one of the emanations of God. Love emanates from God as light emanates from the sun. There can be no lasting goodness, health, peace or joy without love. Hell is the complete separation from God and that would incur also a complete separation from love. Can you imagine what that would be like?

There would be no beauty without love. There would be no light. There would be no life because life itself is an emanation of love. There would be no joy, no peace, nothing of any good whatever. It is hard to imagine when we sit in the midst of the evidence of God's Love.

I get up in the morning and my heart swells with love to such an extent that sometimes I think I am going to just explode in a zillion atoms of pulsating, humming love, and all because my soul is responding to what the Father has revealed of Himself to me.

The sun comes up over the hill and colors the sky, magnificently, as the multi-colored birds begin singing their grateful response. The sun glistens on the droplets of dew quivering on the geniously crafted flowers just beyond the patio and I become so full of adoration for Him, Who has made all this for our enjoyment, that I, sometimes, shout at the top of my voice, "PRAISE THE LORD!" I never get tired of His world. I can't ever take it for granted. The wild cherry trees, laden with flowers, pour an intoxicating incense into the air to rise as a sweet savor before His Throne. I am reminded of His unending love.

The recognition of His love and our response to it is the first move toward the unfolding of the spiritual consciousness within man. This is a progressive state which culminates in the transfiguration.

Solomon, the man of peace, was ordained of God to build the temple of Jerusalem. Solomon was strengthened in his kingdom and the Lord his God was with him, and magnified him.

David was beloved of God, but he was a man of war. He had spilled the blood of many, and because of this, he could not build the temple of God. God wanted a man with clean hands, a man of peace, and thus was Solomon chosen for this momentous occupation.

We are told that he was strengthened in his kingdom, which is to say, he had control over the carnal nature more than any other man of his day. Solomon walked with the God of his fathers and magnified the Spirit of God through his entire being.

He " . . . *went to the high place that was at Gibeon; for there was the tabernacle of the congregation of God, which Moses the servant of the Lord, had made in the wilderness.*" (2 Chron. 1:3)

"A high place" means elevated consciousness. Gibeon was a royal city of the Canaanites. The people there had made peace with the Israelites. Eventually, this land was given to the Levites, the spiritual priesthood of Israel.

You may wonder what all this ancient history of the Old Testament has to do with the subject of this writing: it is to bring light to why you are unhealthy and how you are going to get better and stay that way. The answer to every question of life is in the Word of God. The way of escape from the dilemma of man is revealed in the Word. But it is given for *"those who have ears to hear what is spoken unto the church."* (Rev. 2:7 Paraphrased) I am not offering you the teaching of any man, nor some current theology, psychology, teaching, doctrine, affirmation or formula. I have attempted to lead you from the outer . . . where sickness is visible . . . to the innermost parts . . . where sickness begins, so that when you are confronted in the future with any imbalance of any kind, you will seek out the origin and become re-established in our Father, Who grants all prayers in accordance with the desires of our hearts.

In 2 Chronicles Gibeon represents an illumined state of consciousness where man is able to realize his oneness in and with the triune God. This illumination is positively necessary before man can begin work on the temple because, prior to this time, he was able to build only a synagogue (spiritualized intellect) or the outer courts of the Holy Temple.

Now we understand that Solomon was not a perfect man. He was a mortal man with a penchant for the ladies, and in his old age, he lamented, *" . . . Vanity of vanities, all is vanity . . . "* (Ecc. 1:2) in relation to his mortal life. It is understandable that a man with a thousand wives would get terribly depressed at times and consider life not worth living.

When we examine the symbolical characters of the Old Testament who had tremendous callings to live a represented concept which would be an example for all future generations, the one requisite they had was WILLINGNESS TO SERVE. None of them was perfect. Some were foolish at times. Others were often cowardly and faithless. But they were "willing to serve" where they stood. Take note:

One: We can be of service right now if we are willing to turn everything over to His control.

Two: If we are chosen for service we should not get the idea that we have been set apart because we are special or saintly or more spiritual.

To be a vessel of honor, we need to make a "thousand sacrifices" as Solomon did; sacrifices which are a representation of all our personal desires and ideas. Some people think they are ready to build the temple when they go to Gibeon to the tabernacle and say, "Okay, Lord, I am ready. Use me." And the Lord says, "I don't smell the savor of your sacrifices. Have you lit the fire?" And we say, "Sacrifices?

What sacrifices?" And the Lord says, "Well, how about your desire for material goods, that car and house, that job which puts you in the limelight, and didn't you plan on going to Europe and what about that class you are teaching at church, and what about the children? . . ." And we say, "well, on second thought . . . can I come back next year?" Or we may reason, "Lord, didn't I give up smoking and having a beer now and then and movies and hanging out with the crowd at the dance hall and watching television and reading love stories? Won't those sacrifices do?" And the Lord answers, "You have placed diseased animals on the altar before me and I don't want those sacrifices. I didn't give you those things to begin with so why offer them up to me as sacrifice?"

There has to be an earnest desire to have only the presence of the Lord and to count that as gain. You might say, "Yes Lord . . . on second thought . . . I will come back later. I really am not yet ready to have the fruits of the Spirit manifested in my life. I'm going to this really great dinner tomorrow and Martha makes the best pies. . . ."

For nearly seven years, since the loss of my young son, I had purposed that my life would become a blessing to all those whose lives I touched. I made the conscious decision at that time that I was going to learn all that Jesus would have me learn so that I could travel the highway spoken of by Isaiah.

Although my heart and soul have been totally committed to this walk since then, I have had my periods in the desert of Midian and I have been told on several occasions when I

thought I was ready to start up the Mountain Horeb . . .
"One more time around the mountain, Joyce." I have had
periods of testing when it seemed that darkness would all
but encompass me, and I know about the fiery serpents that
bite and sting when one is wandering, alone, in the wilderness.

But inwardly, something has continued to draw, encourage, and inspire me. Even though, many times I have gotten
weary of this sojourn and wept along the side of the road.

But 1969 was one of those years when the way seems clear
in the wilderness. The desert was blooming and the cloud
was before me in the daytime and the pillar of fire by night.

For forty days I followed a "no pleasant bread" fast as
I felt led to do. During that time I stayed close to the Lord
and magnified Him in my life.

On May 5, 1969 just before noon while I was running the
vacuum sweeper in the living room, the Lord spoke to me
and called me to prayer. I listened to the directions given
and wrote them down in my notebook. I was to sit in prayer
or meditation each day at noon and again at midnight, for
one hour, and the Lord would instruct me in what He wanted
me to do. The Lord proved Himself through the Word, for
each direction given had a Scriptural foundation.

After months of reading the Word day and night, it was as
though a bright cloud came down over me and the Lord
showed me many mighty and wonderful things, some of
which I will share with you now – twelve years later. Why so
long? Because the Lord does not want us to teach anything
of which we have only head knowledge. If we teach only
that which we know intellectually, we are likely to make

fools of ourselves. The wisdom of God and His mysteries are given to the spirit of those who seek it. That wisdom must incubate there and be assimilated into every atom of the soul, and at every level of consciousness. It must then be proved at the personality level. Then one can say, "I have been taught of no man, but God has revealed it unto me." It matters not whether a man believes or understands because we then know that he cannot know except God reveal it to him.

Near the end of the forty days, I went on a two-week retreat to the mountains where I was in guarded spiritual company. Never before or since have I known the presence of God as closely and intimately as I did then. This was the mountaintop experience which every believer longs for and I will never be free to share all of what took place within me.

The hour before my departure from this very special place, the Lord spoke to me and said that when I returned home I would be giving the sermon at church and I was to base the text upon John 4:24, *"God is a spirit; and they that worship him must worship him in spirit and in truth."*

I was further told that this would be the prelude to another prophecy which would be fulfilled and, that a woman would be permitted to speak from the pulpit would be a sign of the events to come.

When I returned home I talked, by telephone, with the pastor of our church, giving him a personal testimony of the events of the retreat and the mighty presence of the Lord which was there. The pastor acknowledged what I'd told him but he didn't say anything about my speaking to the assembly. When our telephone conversation ended, I began to wonder if my *word of knowledge* had been of the Spirit of God or whether it was from my own ego.

That Friday evening a violent tornado ravaged our little country village and brought in its wake heavy rains which inundated much of our State of Ohio. Power lines in our village were down for nearly three days. Our pastor had gone to a Christian camp near Columbus to help bring back the youth of our church and became stranded there when the highways became flooded. The elders of the church had almost decided to cancel services for that Sunday when the president of our church council suggested they ask me to give the message.

Saturday night I was seated in the darkened living room of our home, looking toward our large picture window. I was preparing, in my mind, what I would center my message upon in the morning when suddenly the foyer was brightly illuminated!

I looked toward the foyer in utter amazement, thinking, "How in the world did the light go on" when to my eternal surprise, I saw an illuminating Being about seven feet tall moving toward me from the hallway. Instantly, I was enveloped in a great warmth of love and beauty. I gasped in utter astonishment but had not another moment for any kind of thought because just that suddenly the Being was before me. He reached out a hand and touched me in the center of the forehead and spoke to my spirit, *"Thou shalt love the Lord thy God with all thy heart, and with all thy soul, and with all thy mind, and thy neighbor as thyself and spread joy throughout the universe."* Instantly, I was caught up in the Spirit.

With the swiftness of a rushing wind, I was lifted up in the Spirit. Momentarily, I thought I'd been struck by lightening! I should have been afraid, but everything happened so fast that I was caught off guard. My entire being was filled with such joy that I could not be afraid. My heart opened up to love such as I had never known possible. If I had died at that moment the death certificate would have read, "heart failure," but it really would have been spiritual rapture. I heard music playing, filling up all space with melodious strains as if performed by a mighty orchestra. It was more beautiful than anything I had ever heard. I was particularly conscious of the string section. However, now I can only faintly recall this heavenly strain.

During this time, it seemed I'd been moving through space at a tremendous speed. It was as though I was catapulted out of my body with such a tremendous force that I burst right through the top of my head. When I got up so high, I burst out of another body, again and again, until I was no longer speeding through space. Every vestige of "me" had fallen away: the physical body, the emotional body, the mental body, the body of my soul. I seemed to lose my identity as "Joyce," my ego, and my identity as an individual.

When the sense of movement had stopped I had the awareness of a brilliant white light far above, around, and below me. I was in the light and the light was in me. And the light was God. And God was the light! I knew no separateness from Him. My own being, my spirit . . . was endless, boundless; it encompassed all creation and all creation was in me and it was all light. I had no form, no identity, no awareness

of separate individuality. There was neither time, nor space,
no method of thought. I WAS! That is all that I can say. I
was the nothingness which is the All! Yet it was not an empty nothingness. It was a nothingness which was fertile with
everything, for everything was contained within it.

Here, on this earth, we can experience on thing at one
time. If we listen to music, we cannot be fully absorbed
in painting a sunset. But in the nothingness of God which
is all encompassing I could feel the majesty of the *Painted
Desert* and *Niagara Falls* and the *Texas prairies* all at once.

I descended from that place where I had been one with God,
and I knew myself to be in God, but I had individuality as a
separate spirit. I had to descend in consciousness in order to
know this individuality and it was an overwhelmingly sad feeling of great loss. It was a lowering from that high place where
a moment before I had dwelt as a mere cell in the body of God.

At this lower level of consciousness, I sensed my spirit,
and realized that I had form even as the Being who had
brought me to this place had form. The form was glowing
and iridescent, luminous and perfect. It was then that I knew
that this was my natural state of being – the Image of God
in which I had been originally created. I realized that any
other thought I had ever held of myself was a lie perpetrated
by the *enemy* to keep me in bondage to the world of carnal
flesh. I was aware that, at this level of being, I, my natural
self, was beyond sin and error, and that this place of spirit
was truly a place of perfection – not because only the perfect are permitted to dwell there, but because sin and error
and imperfection have been completely washed away by the

blood of the *Perfect Sacrifice.*

Then I was brought from the place of spirit to the plane of soul and I became aware of an even greater chasm between my two levels of consciousness. The Great Light, in which I had just a moment before been immersed, had dimmed, and another great wave of sadness swept over me as I realized the gulf between my Father and I was growing. Now I was able to be objective, subjective, and feel what was going on about me. A moment before, at the level of spirit, I was cognizant. There was no natural thinking process. I had been in the mind of God and the mind of God had been in me. I knew what God knew and God knew what I knew and there was no difference. But at the level of soul, I did not know what God knew. Already the door between the spirit mind and the soul mind had been closed. I could remember that I had known, but I could not remember what I had known. I was disdained at such a tremendous reduction in stature and being — such a limitation of mind and feeling and aware- ness — such a closing in on me of the world I had glimpsed into just a moment before. How narrow and dark it seemed compared to where I just had been. How heavy and burden- some was the limited *soul body* in which I now had to ex- press myself.

As pure soul being, I was aware that I stood in the *Great Divide,* bridging the worlds of my spirit and my ego. I was aware of both of the great opposing forces working upon my nature; one which drew me forcefully and sweetly toward the glories of heaven and the other which tore at me like the swirling waters of a whirlpool to bring me back to the lure of the earth and mortal body.

My soul became burdened with a grief such as I had never known. I struggled to keep alive, in memory, all the glories of *Divine Liberation* which I had been shown in my Father's house. But, even as I struggled, I could feel that I was succumbing to the drawing force of the earth and to my mortal body. I descended into matter with a heavy feeling of sorrow because that quick return to the native land of my spirit had been far too brief, and I knew that nothing this side of heaven would ever, so completely, fill me again.

In a flash, I was back with my mortal body, still seated in an upright position on the davenport, still hugging my knees to my chest as I had been when the Being first appeared. The house was darkened once more. The village on the other side of the lake was still cloaked in utter blackness. My children were still sleeping peacefully in their beds. The forms of the furniture in the darkened living room still looked the same. There was no visible evidence that this visitation had ever taken place. . . . I would wonder, for many years, why I had had this supernatural experience.

But one thing was accomplished which nothing on this earth could change. Those brief moments of being in the presence of Almighty God have left their mark on me. God has hidden something within my heart which makes me His possession. I have no other desire than to serve Him. I know, above all else, that it is the desire of every human to come to self-realization, or self-awareness, so that he can know the sacred treasure living within him. Once we see, with our spiritual eyes, that we are made in the Image of

God, we will willingly give up all these occupations we have invented to assuage our discomfort.

You are not just a flesh and blood body inhabited by a self-centered ego which selfishly procrastinates and balks before the insistent call of our Lord. What earth-bound people are struggling to hold onto isn't even real. It is all part of the Satanic lie which Adam and Eve accepted without question and bequethed to all these following generations. We have accepted the lie and believed the delusion that we are separated from God when in fact and truth, we have never left Him, nor had He left us. We are as much in Him as the fish are in the ocean. But is the fish anymore aware of the sea than we are of the Father? *"I live, and move, and have my being in God who has made me."* (Acts 17:28 Paraphrased)

And, because we have forgotten that we are in God, and He is in us, we believe what we see through our senses . . . that we are in this world and the world is in us. We have *"borne the image of the earthy"* (1 Cor. 15:9 Paraphrased), and as such, we inherit all the curses and woes laid upon the earth. We may say that we are now new creatures in Christ, and, although this is true, we understand this only inellectually. It is not yet imprinted upon every cell of our body, mind, soul and spirit. And, until it is, the truths which Jesus taught us, the affirmations and promises given to us as children of God, remain as intellectual gems. We have not *appropriated* them as our own. Instead, we have appropriated the belief in sickness, tribulation, poverty, war, famine, pestilence and death. *This* is what is written upon every cell of our entire nature. And, as long as it is, we will have to deal with suffering and tribulation as does the rest of the world. That is, until we receive the mind of Christ.

"But when that which is perfect is come, then that which is in part shall be done away." (1 Cor. 13:10) Scripture tells us that those who waited for the coming of the Holy Spirit, in the *Upper Room,* received the fullness of the mind of Christ. They had an experience which we have not had. If we say that the experience they had was only for them and for that time, then, we would be limiting God and His ability to work through us. He was able to work through the apostles, in a greater way, because of the experience they had in the *Upper Room.* There is more to come! Jesus said we would do *greater* works than He did. We need to pray for a greater revelation of God's Word. We need to *appropriate the power* in order to do the work which remains to be done. *"And that knowing the time, that now it is high time to awake out of sleep: for now is our salvation nearer than when we believed."* (Rom. 13:11)

The sleep from which we must awaken is the belief that this world of sense consciousness and materiality is our real world. Sitting there with this book in your hand, this world seems as real as can be. And, as I work here in my dining room, looking out into the backyard at the few lingering patches of snow, the barren trees at the top of the hill and the little juncos picking at crumbs on the patio, I, too, am in a real world. Physically, I am very warm, and I get a little pain over my right eye every once in a while, and, in the background, the kitchen faucet is monotonously dripping.

This world seems just as real to me as it does to you. The part that isn't real, my friends, is the feeling you and I have right now that God is far away through time and space; that we cannot know Him until we "get to heaven," and that all the promises, rewards, joys and glories have to wait until then.

For a very long time, I did not know what the Lord intended when He sent one of His messengers to reveal this to me. I pondered it, prayed over it, questioned it, and sought for an answer. After a time, I just folded up the memory of the experience and stored it away with "herbs and aloes." I went on about my life — down here in the wilderness area. Then I had another desert experience and I spent two and a half years there, which isn't such a very long time, but it seemed endless. And during that time, I was tested almost to the end of my endurance, confronted with an experience similar to Job's, minus the boils. Everything in this world that I held of value was taken away. Everything. And the voice of wickedness tempted, saying, "Curse God and die." But I would not, because I know God. I know Him personally. I know His nature and I know His love. And I know, beyond a shadow of a doubt, throughout every fiber of my being, that whatever befalls me in life, it cannot conquer me. No matter what the cause of the affliction, the tribulation, the sorrow . . . *God is always triumphant in my life and He takes every boulder that would fall on me and makes it a stepping stone to Him!*

There followed two and a half more years in the desert, watching over the flocks, knowing that God was there but I could not reach Him because I had to tend the sheep. I had to weigh, and judge and evaluate. I had to understand, analyze and assimilate. I had to "number the sheep."

And when it was God's time, He allowed me to understand both my stay in the desert and my trip to the mountaintop. And all that had been taken away was given back and added to, good measure, filled up, pressed down and running over.

The Father wants you to know that you don't have to wait until His return to earth to come nigh unto Him. You don't have to wait until you die and "go to heaven." You don't have to be perfect or special. He wants to give you your inheritance in Canaan and He wants you to start to work on the temple. He wants you to come into the Holy of Holies.

Our Father reminds us that Jesus rent the veil of the Holy of Holies so that it is no longer necessary to have a high priest to intercede for us. He invites us to meet with Him. He makes this message available in these latter days through many, like myself, who have no special attributes whatever that would give them special honor. He has chosen the foolish to confound the wise of this world.

He has shown me, through my supernatural experience, that the kingdom of God is within. Although, through this memorable experience, it seemed that I had travelled to distant planets far out in space, I had gone no where but within!

I had been shown the other parts of myself which, before that time, I had not known existed. I thought I knew all there was of me, because I had always been an introspective, analytical person. But I was shown that all that I knew of me was my conscious intellectual self and a surface introduction to my soul. I had not even begun to tap all the reserve of wisdom, power, ability and spiritual gifts which are part of my nature in Christ.

I know, with a deep inner spiritual knowing, that which is true of me is true of you, for we are alike. We are His, and we are made like Him. I understand what Paul meant when he said that when we see Him we shall know Him for we shall be like Him. Yes, we will. When we have cast off this soiled garment of carnality and permit the glorious beauty of Christ to appear in us, we shall be like Him!

II

Are You Possessing The Land?

"For what man knoweth the things of a man, save the spirit of man which is in him? even so the things of God knoweth no man, but the spirit of God. . . . that we might know the things that are freely given to us of God. Which things also we speak, not in the words which man's wisdom teacheth, but which the Holy Ghost teacheth; comparing spiritual things with spiritual. But the natural man receiveth not the things of the Spirit of God: for they are foolishness unto him: neither can he know them, because they are spiritually discerned. But he that is spiritual judgeth all things, yet he himself is judged of no man. For who hath known the mind of the Lord, that he may instruct him? But we have the mind of Christ." (1 Cor. 2:11-16)

Can we claim, . . . at the level of consciousness where 99% of us function on a day-to-day basis, that we have the mind of Christ? Are we demonstrating those attributes which are of Christ or of the sense-conscious man? Do we manifest "the spirit of counsel and might, the spirit of knowledge"?

Do we "know all things"? Do we have hid within "all the treasures of wisdom and knowledge"? Are all things delivered unto us of the Father? Do we have "counsel and sound wisdom, understanding, strength"? Do we "know all men"? Can we honestly say with Him, ". . . *I seek not mine own will, but the will of the father which hath sent me."* (John 5:30)

I began the research for this book when I observed born-again believers, with a good measure of faith, believing for things which did not come to pass. They prayed, claimed the promise, stood on the Word, . . . did everything as was prescribed in Scriptures, and yet the manifestation did not take place.

It was the conflict between what was believed and what took place that began my introspective study of the Scripture, much prayer and fasting, and weeks of seeking His annointing. This is what I found, . . . we do not yet have the mind of Christ. The mind of Christ is available to us. All that the Son is heir to, we have inherited through Him, for we are in Him and He is in us. He took us unto Himself when He came to this earth to be Saviour and Redeemer of mankind. He opened His heart and closed it around all of us. And, although we cannot grasp the magnanimity of that truth, because it is beyond our finite minds, we can accept in faith that it is so. What we have, as we abound in faith and the Word, is an intellectual conscious acknowledgement of the mind of Christ. We do not have the fullness of the mind of Christ. If we did, we would be performing the miracles we believe are possible. We have the faith to raise the dead, but we do not have the power! And we know that the word says, " . . . *All power is given unto me in heaven and in earth.* " (Matt. 28:18) *"If ye abide in me, and my words abide in you, ye shall ask what ye will, and it shall be done unto you."* (John 15:7) *"And whatsoever ye shall ask in my name, that will I do, that the Father may be glorified in the Son."* (John 14:13)

"Abide in me. . . . " What does it mean? It obviously would have to mean more than what we are presently doing with our daily prayers and Bible reading, memory Scripture, prayer meetings and church fellowship.

Webster defines *abide* as: To take up one's abode; to reside. To be prepared for; to await; be able to endure or sustain; remain firm under; to tolerate, adhere to, maintain; remain faithful; satisfied with.

"Abide in me, . . . " (John 15:4) says the Lord. *"Take up your abode in me, reside in me, be prepared for me, await me, be able to endure for me, remain firm under me, tolerate me, adhere to me, maintain me, remain faithful to me; be satisfied with me."* (Paraphrased) The Greek word for abide is *meno* which translates *"unbroken communion."*

In the last chapter it was explained that, spiritually, we do abide in Christ. The difficulty is that we do not abide in *our* spirit. Only as we meet the requirement of abiding in our spirit, with unbroken communion with Him, can we ask whatever we will in His name and it shall be done unto us. The reason is that the natural man and the spiritual man are functioning on two different planes of expression. The spiritual man can function in the natural realm but the nat-

ural man cannot function in the spiritual realm. And even
the most sincere among us function out of the natural 99%
of the time, and only on special occasions do we rise to
the *spiritual plane.*

During the initial drafting of this chapter, the problem of
functioning out of the spirit became foremost to me. I
wanted to tell you what was right and true and I didn't know
how, because I couldn't solve the problem for myself. How
do we function out of the spirit? How do we abide in Him
that whatsoever we ask shall be done? The Lord answered all
my questions at one time and in a single experience.

My eighteen-year old son, Michael, was playing baseball
with the church team. He was getting ready to leave for a
game one Wednesday evening. I was standing at the top of
the stairs of our house, watching him go down to the car of
another young man who also played on the team. As I
watched these two clean-cut, sincere Christian boys leave for
the game, I was suddenly overwhelmed with a feeling that
something was going to happen while they were gone that
evening. I immediately began praying in the Spirit and
visualizing them surrounded by the protection of God's
love. I prayed until I felt peace in my heart.

An hour or so later, I was walking into the church for our
Wednesday evening prayer meeting and Bible Study. Just
as I walked through the door, our pastor beckoned me to
his office saying, "Mike's been hurt playing baseball and is
at the hospital!" Immediately, instantaneously, I was taken
up in the Spirit. It was as if a giant vacuum cleaner literally
sucked my consciousness up onto a higher plane. I was no

longer sitting in the church office. I was in the kingdom of God. There was a glorious light shining all about me. There was peace. There was assurance. There was joy. There was calm. I prayed in the Spirit, praising God for His majesty and glory. I didn't have my mind on Michael or hospital or injury or fear or trouble. That is because in the kingdom of God, none of these things exist. There is only GOOD in the kingdom of God. There could be no turning of my mind in the spiritual realm because there was nothing else but God.

My pastor handed me the telephone and I felt assured that everything was alright and that I was not needed there. The mother of the other young man was standing in my place and, since she also is a born-again Christian, I felt very secure that the Lord was in charge of everything. I was about to go in to the prayer meeting when the Spirit spoke to my heart and told me to go, at once, to the hospital.

Shortly after arriving there, I discovered why the Spirit of God wanted me at the hospital. (This was to be an unforgettable teaching session).

My son had been playing the position of catcher that evening and when the second man on the other team was up to bat, as a lefthanded hitter, he swung around with the bat and hit my son on the side of the head. Michael hit the ground under the impact, the side of his head near the temple being split open, but he bounced back up immediately, barely stunned! The fellows on our team rushed to his side, made a circle around him, layed hands upon him and began praying. They were quite a visible witness to the other team by their faith and peace in the Lord.

When I arrived at the emergency room of the hospital, the nurses permitted me to go to my son's side. With a Bible in my hand, I entered his room and began to pray.

Soon the stitches were in place and Michael was in the process of being released. But as he was about to sign the release papers, he went into shock and fell, like a tree, against the terrazo floor! Immediately, he started going into convulsion. But just as quickly, I was down on the floor beside him, laying hands on him, binding the enemy and praying in the Spirit! The doctors and nurses let me alone until I was finished and Michael was slowly coming back to himself! Then they lifted him onto a gurney and called for a neurosurgeon and a series of catscan x-rays.

I was there most of the night but even after all those hours, I didn't get weary and I never feared. I knew deep inside of me that all was well. Two days later, Michael was released from the hospital and, as believed, there was nothing serious wrong with him. And I had learned a marvelous lesson — first hand.

At our present level of spiritual development and commitment, we can operate out of the spirit consciousness WHEN GOD WILLS IT! *I* hadn't immediately changed levels of operation when I heard the news of my son's injury. I hadn't done it because I didn't know how. I was willing to be used as a channel for healing, and since God wanted my son to be well, He chose to use me. God brought about the conditions, gave me foreknowledge, impressed me to be "prayed up" even before the accident accured. He gave me boldness to be able to do what needed to be done at the hospital. He empowered me to act as Jesus would have acted. That is something I couldn't have done by my own strength. In fact, my son was reluctant to have me find out about his accident, because he was expecting that I would act out of the old (dead) natural self which he remembered from his childhood days. He knew better than anyone that "Mom" was under the power of the Holy Spirit. And it was glorious to be so fully possessed of Him.

John 1:6-9 says, *"There was a man sent from God, whose name was John. The same came for a witness, to bear witness of the Light, that all men through him might believe. He was not that Light, but was sent to bear witness of that Light. That was the true Light, which lighteth every man that cometh into the world."* John was speaking, of course, of Jesus Christ.

Jesus was the *Incarnate Word* and He was the *Light.* And we are asked to abide in this *Light,* which is Christ. And because we were created in the image and likeness of God, the true *Light* of Christ has been placed in every man that cometh into the world.

Our physical bodies are composed of countless atoms, aggregated and sustained by the superconscious mind of the individual acting in cooperation with *Divine Mind.* Each miniscule atom is an entire replica of our solar system, its tiny protons, neutrons and electrons representing planets which are rotating around a nucleus equivalent to the sun. Each atom which makes up a solid has an electrical center which can bring forth a manifestation of an attribute of the invisible spiritual realm, giving scientific proof of the omnipresence of the Spirit of God!

As long as the atom remains undisturbed, the electrons go on revolving just as the earth revolves, and no energy is let off or taken in. But, if some outside force acts upon the atom, the electron is forced to change its orbit. If the orbit is changed to a smaller orbit, thereby rotating faster, radiant energy called quantum is given off, producing light, color and sound, each of which is synchronized on a spectrum scale. In this last century, man has discovered the hidden forces of nature and begun using them to improve our physical life with the use of electricity, radio waves, x-rays, radar, sonic impulses and gamma rays. We are only a step away from understanding how to harness and use these energies to improve our spiritual life as well.

Energy and power are synonymous, and energy produces light. A few years ago some researchers in a laboratory made an accidental discovery. In observing the blood sample of a certain patient, a very reverant minister, they noted something unusual about his blood cell. Under a high-powered microscope lens it appeared that the nucleus of the cell was light. Excited by the discovery the researchers began collecting blood samples of a cross-section of society. Hundreds of tests supported the theory that morally upright, ethical people had varying degrees of light within the cell. Highly devotional and "spiritual" people had a marked increase in the amount of light within the cell. Blood samples drawn from convicts on death row, in one prison, showed no light whatever in their blood samples. Here was startling evidence — but what did it indicate?

Many tests and investigations eventually led the researchers to this conclusion: light in the blood cell is produced by breath. When one is relaxed and in harmony with himself and his fellow man, he breathes deeply, drawing in a fresh supply of oxygen with every inhalation. The oxygen feeds the entire blood system, hence the entire body, with not only the physical properties needed for the sustenance of life, but also with spiritual properties.

Persons who consciously apply themselves to a higher degree of spirituality quite often engage in a program of deep diaphramatic breathing as part of their meditation and contemplation. Their reward is a higher degree of light in the physical system which feeds the invisible spiritual qualities into the mind and the emotional nature as well.

Conversely, it was discovered that when a person is even considering acting out of accord with the highest moral and ethical value he knows he immediately begins a shallow breathing pattern which does not feed the body the physical properties which are essential but cheats the soul and spiritual bodies as well.

Many people, including doctors, recognize the benefits of deep rhythmic breathings as a tonic for stress. It is also advisable for insomniacs and has been invaluable to the mentally and emotionally disturbed. But the simple, automatic function of breathing is far more important to us than previously imagined.

We already have agreed that man is a trinity: a spirit, having an individualized soul which functions through a physical body. Yet even this explanation is incomplete for both the soul and the body are multifarious in nature and able to express themselves, separately and simultaneously, and in different forms.

An example of the complexity of the mind is the information available to scientists through the use of biofeedback machines. Different levels of consciousness or mind activities are discernable and measurable with this modern equipment. The machine indicates when the person has entered into another state of consciousness, from beta (objective) to alpha (subjective) to theta (dream) and finally into the delta state which indicates life in another dimension. Even though we generally are unaware of the various levels of consciousness, we each pass through all of them each time we fall asleep and each time we awaken. We are governed by various principles which have different vehicles of expression. They are: 1. Spirit; 2. Superconscious Mind; 3. Soul; 4. Subconscious Mind; 5. Intellect; 6. Physical Body; 7. Vital Force (or breath of God).

It is the vital force or the breath of God which gives life to the physical and which holds together the spirit, soul, and body. When the vital force is withdrawn, the soul leaves the body and that which we call "death" ensues because the body will quickly decay once the vital force is withdrawn.

The breath of God is the creative substance from which all things are made and without it is nothing that is made. The breath of God is everywhere; in, around, and through all creation. It is creative energy, a "breathing out" of God with the Word which speaks all creation into form. It was the breath of God expelling the words *"Let there be . . . "* (Gen. 1:3) which called the atoms abounding in space to cohese and take on the materialized form visualized in the mind of God.

Although the breath of God is in all matter, it is not matter. Rather, it is the energy which animates all matter. The breath of God is potent with energy which can be utilized and directed as tremendous power. It can be made to accomplish a variety of things.

Power produces heat and light. The greater the power, the more intense the heat and the brighter the light. Solar energy is the best example we have visibly available.

The breath of God can be consciously used by us to produce energy, power, heat and light. This energy can be used for healing, restoration of one's physical body, to illuminate and increase one's ability to retain knowledge, to increase one's creative inspiration, to overcome the cravings of the flesh toward harmful habits, to lower one's pulse or blood pressure, to calm anxiety and nervousness, and to feed a weakened soul which has been starved of the Light of the Word.

The breath of God is in the air but it is neither air nor one of its chemical constituents. It is taken into the body along with the air we breathe, but it is not oxygen.

Moses knew the difference between the atmospheric air and the breath of God contained within it. He speaks of "neshemet ruach chayim" which means "the breath of the spirit of life." The Hebrew word "neshemet" means the ordinary breath of air. "Chayim" means life; while the word "ruach" means the "spirit of life." Therefore, we see that the ordinary and primary act of simply breathing in imparts to us more than the mere physiological benefit of taking in oxygen necessary to life. We are also taking in the breath of God which sustains and vitalizes our life. The spirit and soul of man does not need oxygen in order to live but they do need the breath of God.

How few of us realize that by consciously absorbing the breath of God along with every intake of oxygen we can increase the light within our soul bodies and awaken higher spiritual awareness.

The breath of God is truly the balm of Gilead. When we recognize and give credit to God as the source of all our good we can utilize this vital energy at a higher level — to literally transform water into wine. We are all using the breath of God in every thing we do. But, it can be no more than an impotent substance, such as plain water, when it is used without the exercising of the will. When we act in cooperation with God as co-creator with Him, acknowledging Him and speaking forth the Word of creation in the name of Jesus, this vital force, which is overlooked and taken for granted by the multitudes, suddenly becomes charged with a higher degree of energy. We have called forth power from on high and the water is turned to wine! This was the first miracle of Jesus and it can be the first miracle for us when we accept the authority given us by Christ — to use His name to do all the works He did!

The vital force or the breath of God abounds in us, yet we waste it as if it were no more than stagnant water. We fluster about, chewing our nails, jiggling our feet, twisting our fingers. We call this the result of nervous energy. It is an abundance of the vital force stored in the ganglion and nerve centers of our bodies which we do not know how to use properly! If we used our wills to direct this abundant energy to the higher nerve centers in our bodies, we would increase our mental powers, we would have God's power behind our prayers, we would increase the strength of the inner man by feeding him upon the "Bread of Life" . . . (another name for the vital force) and we would build a reservoir of power for the laying on of hands!

What is the sense of laying hands on another unless we are imparting a healing touch to that person? If there is no healing power in our hands what have we availed by touching them? If the healing power is there in your hands, you know it! Whenever you are a channel for power from on high, you know it! Do you think it possible that God could use you or visit you mightily with His Spirit and you not feel totally different than when you are doing the dishes or greasing the car? Incredible!

Several years ago we had a mother cat who had a litter of kittens. They had gone beyond the weaning stage and we hadn't found homes for all of them. We had quite a houseful of precious little furry babies running around, and I loved every one of them. One afternoon I was busy in the kitchen, preparing dinner, when the little four-year old girl next door walked into the living room looking for my children who hadn't yet come home from school. When the little girl got ready to leave, the kittens apparently tried to follow her, and knowing I didn't want them outside, she quickly shut the door and squeezed my favorite kitten in the door. Frightened by what she had done, she ran off home without telling me about the kitten. It was nearly two hours later before my children came home and when they did I was alarmed by these horrible screams from all four of them.

Tearfully, they came into the kitchen carrying the limp body of the little white kitten and my son, Chucky, cried, "Mommy, *do something!*"

The little kitten looked dead. It's glassy eyes were frozen in an unblinking stare, a foul-smelling substance had oozed from its mouth, nose and rectum and its little body had not a faint glimmer of life in it. But my children were looking to me to *"do something!"*

I didn't think or reason or analyze. My heart was moved by my children's faith in my prayers and my spirit was moved by the need of that precious creature. I took it in my hands and stood before the window (which was closed), held its little body up toward heaven, and prayed God to heal that animal and bring life back to it.

At 3:30 p.m. that afternoon, the presence of Almighty God, in answer to a mother's prayers for the sake of the faith of her children, came down upon that little village and entered into our house!

Momentarily, my body was filled with a tremendous jolt of energy which was akin to electrical shock and the light of God was brilliant all around us. I felt my hands tremble under the power of so great a force. Suddenly, I heard a faint little "mew" and the kitten stirred in my hands and lifted its head. It was back among the living!

Two hours later, when their father came home from

work, everything was back to normal. However, as soon as he stepped into the kitchen he stopped and said, "What happened here?" Two hours later, you see, our kitchen was still charged with the supernatural power from on high!

Sincere Christians, who want to be of service to God but who have no directive to follow, can wander around, aimlessly, and never be able to bring about the condition they desire where they are a *"vessel of honor in the household of the Lord."* (1 Chron. 28:13 Paraphrased) They have faith in the substance of things hoped for yet unseen, but sooner or later, those unseen things should materialize. They do not need to go on, forever, claiming that something exists when they don't see it. The time should come when they can see that what they hoped for IS there.

The other evening, several people at a church service went forward, desiring to receive the Holy Spirit. I felt the annointing of the Spirit upon me and the power flowing into my body and out of my hands. I felt *inner directed* to go forward and direct the power to a young lady who wanted to receive. A man came up behind me and, wanting to help, laid his hand on me. The vital force went out of me into him. People can also do this when they want to heal someone. They don't know how to receive the power of life through the breath of God because they don't know about it. They lay hands on someone who is in a weakened condition and end up making that person weaker. They are sincere but they don't know what they are doing!

Water is symbolic of instability. Our use of the vital force, without spiritualized consciousness of it and what it does, is unstable. It may be there for us to use at one time and devoid of us at another time. It may depend upon our mental or emotional condition or whether we are rested or exhausted. We can have a moment of anger or impatience and dissipate all the vital force we have stored for a week. We can waste the vital force through meaningless chatter, needless restlessness, too much physical activity, or allowing the mind to jump nervously from one thing to another. Do you think it was so with Jesus? Hardly! When someone had a need, the breath of God was available to Him to use to meet every need.

Wine symbolizes the spiritual vitality which is generated through a conscious link (the marriage at Cana) established between the soul and body acting in one accord. When this mystical marriage takes place between the personality and the soul, no longer are we a kingdom divided which shall crumble and fall. Now the best wine which was saved until the last is brought forth so that all may drink their fill. We begin to appropriate the vitalized breath of God.

The vital force, which has been stored in the nerve centers of the body, becomes activated with new life, and the soul actually begins singing within us. There comes a time when a gentle humming begins in the area of the larnyx. *Cana means place of the reeds and this in itself represents the larnyx where our "speaking reeds" are contained.* When we feel this activity of the spiritualized vital force we *know* that we can speak forth the words of power. And when we misuse that power, it will work against us to bring about disharmony and discordance within our physical vehicle in the form of sore throat, laryngitis, thyroid imbalances.

By the same token, we can consciously increase the vital force in any one of the nerve centers to increase the power of that attribute. These areas are all represented by the stone pots which were used by Jesus to hold the water which was changed into wine.

For instance, if we draw in the breath of God and consciously direct this vital force to the throat area, we can build and increase the power contained within the body. Or we can direct the vital energy to the heart and increase the force of divine love within ourselves. By directing the vital force to the center in the forehead, we increase the power of intuition, an attribute of the soul. And by directing the breath of God to Golgotha, the place of the skull (at the top of the head), the mind of Christ can be lifted up in us.

"The Spirit of God hath made me, and the breath of the Almighty hath given me life." (Job 33:4) *"By the word of the Lord were the heavens made; and all the host of them by the breath of his mouth."* (Psa. 33:6) (God) *"Neither is worshipped with men's hands, as though he needed any thing, seeing he giveth to all life, and breath, and all things; And hath made of one blood all nations of men for to dwell on all the face of the earth, and hath determined the times before appointed, and the bounds of their habitation; That they should seek the Lord, if haply they might feel after him, and find him, though he be not far from every one of us: For in Him we live, and move, and have our being; . . . "* (Acts 17:25-28)

The mind of Christ is more than superman intelligence. The highest genius among mankind is nonetheless a man.

Possessing such genius does not make him a Christ. Jesus had the mind of Christ yet it is not His superior intelligence for which he is remembered and revered. It is His power! And that power is the result of divine love, wisdom and light.

We live and move and have our being in this power. Our spirits are even now partaking of the love, wisdom and light which is Christ. If we could rise in prayer at this moment to that level of Christ, we would be cognizant of the attributes of the *Divine Mind.* We fail in manifesting the power which Jesus said is given to us from on high because: 1. we have not elevated our consciousness to perceive the mind of Christ and 2. if we have perceived or experienced the superconsciousness and its inherent union with the mind of Christ, we have not been able to bring that power down to the mortal level. And, although we might wish to bring this power down to the mortal level, only a few people are able to accomplish it.

The mind of Christ is more than faith. Mortals need faith because they are still in the position of hoping for that which they have not yet seen. The mind of Christ is more than positive thinking, righteous decree or good confession. The mind of Christ is more than a readiness to recite Scripture verbatim. These are devices needed to spiritualize the intellect of mortal man. And while the spiritualization of man's mind is a prerequisite to knowing about God, it cannot supplant KNOWING GOD. Thinking about the mind of Christ does not make us KNOW Him.

Thinking what we believe are the thoughts of the Christ Mind is still an activity of our own intellect, for the mind of

Christ is the absence of thought. It is the I AM THAT I AM. We cannot be that I AM until we have *come into* this mind of Christ. You can stand on the uttermost precipice of the highest mountain in the world, but you will still be unable to touch heaven, because they are in two different realms. One is physical; the other is spiritual. So it is with the intellect of man and the mind of Christ.

Our western culture preordains us to the limitations of intellect. *Adhering to a "Greek-mindedness" of concrete, rational thought, we have nearly enshrined the false god of intellect, oblivious to the fact that man's greatest mental achievement is foolishness in the light of the wisdom of God.*

On the other hand, the oriental mind of abstract, subjective awareness *intuits* that the knower can never be on equal par with the KNOWN. It is the abstract thought, able to move beyond the confines of organized mental form, which is able to flow toward the mind of Christ. Those who were responsible for giving us the bedrock of Judaic-Christian revelation *had* to be those of contemplative, subjective conditioning or they would never have been able to receive the direction of an invisible God. And here we are, Greek-minded intellectuals, trying to make subjective experiences make sense to our deductive mental faculties. Oh, the pride of man!

If we are to achieve all that Jesus taught us we will have to be willing to lay aside our preconceived notions, our necessity to "understand," our preoccupation with "things making sense," our stranglehold upon that which we believe makes us different from the creatures around us . . . our thoughts . . . and just wait upon the Lord — *Ask, Seek, Knock.* It won't come in a moment . . . although the experience itself may come suddenly and without expectation. After a constant and consistent straining of the higher mortal mind motivated by the sincere praise, worship and service of the soul, there will be a sudden tearing asunder of the veil which keeps the "holy of holies" hidden from view. Suddenly the light of Christ will stream forth into the consciousness, flooding the entire inner man, filling him with that "joy unspeakable and full of glory." This light is real and it is visible. The one who has this light revealed to him knows that he has it. He feels it coming into his consciousness, he sees it within when he closes his eyes and he feels when the power of the light goes out from him. And this light is available to everyone who seeks it.

He who seeks will find. It is then that a person becomes aware of a new dimension to his being. Forces and energies previously unknown to him become as common as the hair on his head. And the mind of Christ will influence the mortal or conscious mind in an abstract manner, filling it with wisdom, inspiration, creativity and revelation. The mind of Christ will add power to the concentrated directed thought of the conscious mind. This power from on high is not a *concept* of something invisible. It is a real, observable, detectable energy unlike any physical energy known to man outside of Christ. The possessor of this power knows when it is flowing in his body, because he can feel it just as surely as he can feel his heart beating and his lungs drawing in and expelling air. He knows when this power goes out of him and the point to which it is going. Sometimes he can exercise his will to direct this power where he wants it to go. First we must be made ready to receive this power.

This is the work of the Holy Spirit — quickening the idea born in the intellect of man and transmitting it to spiritual consciousness in order that it can affect our outer domain. Our prayers, therefore, must work at the spiritual level first or there will be no change in the manifested realm of the physical.

"Let this mind be in you, which was also in Christ Jesus:" (Phil. 2:5) is a progressive work which begins with spiritual discernment. This is shown us in the development of the life of Solomon and the Children of Israel which is symbolic of the path of development we, too, must take.

Solomon (Solar Man or Man of Light) was appointed *". . . to build the house of the Lord, and his own house . . . "* (1 Kings 9:15) And he was to be ruler over Israel. But before there was a king, there was a judge.

Spiritual discernment is judge of the land. "But he that is spiritual judgeth all things, yet he himself is judged of no man." The process of judging and choosing begins at the earliest stage of our spiritual development. It is the developing of the conscience which later becomes the *"inner voice."* Through this development of spiritual discernment man learns to choose that which brings him into peaceful harmony with the Creator and to abandon those actions and attitudes which cause discord.

By eliminating negative or destructive thought processes and building up thought patterns of devotion, praise, and service, we develop a receptivity to the Spirit of God. When we are in crisis or chaos we are then able to "hear" His still, small voice speaking to us.

This *inner voice* which brings inspiration and holy thoughts to the consciousness of man will bring also that which is necessary for his deliverance from the bondage of duality and error.

There is no surer teacher than the *inner voice* who gives that which is necessary for us as individuals; leading and guiding in a manner that no mortal, however illumined, could ever do.

It is the *inner voice* which judges that no religious movement, nor man-made creeds and doctrines can supply that which is needed for man to *"put on the fullness of Christ."* (Rom. 13:14 Paraphrased) The cleansing which must take place within is the work of the Holy Spirit in us. He cannot bring us to all truth and sanctification if we do not allow Him to work in this manner. Yet the inside of the plate must be cleaned that we be clean all over for *" . . . when he shall appear, we shall be like him; . . . "* (1 John 3:2) *"And every man that hath this hope in him purifieth himself, even as he is pure."* (1 John 3:3)

There is no short cut to letting the mind of Christ be in you. We cannot get in by the back door. Methods and procedures mentioned here have been used by those of different religious persuasions. Some of them are highly developed, spiritually disciplined people of impeccable motivation and habit. Yet they do not have the power from on high. Nor do they have the mind of Christ. They have their own disciplined spirituality which avails them nothing because he who would come unto the Father *must* come through Christ!

In these latter days, when the Holy Spirit of God is being poured out upon all flesh, many are being offered the opportunity to come up onto higher ground than was possible in ages past. It is difficult to cut ourselves loose from the things of this world in order to become spiritually pure. But it is not impossible. I have known many persons involved in Eastern religions who have achieved a high degree of physical and emotional purity. They have cleansed the mind, emotions and body of all carnal desire with discipline and execution of will. They have achieved this high level of mortal purity and have through meditation achieved a high degree of inner stability. But because they are not born-again, they remain flesh-and-blood, which cannot inherit spiritual things. Imagine what we could accomplish for the glory of Jesus Christ if we Christians were as devoted to our Lord as they are to their statutes.

We who have been baptized into the Body of Christ have been given every weapon necessary to overcome, not only temptation, but sin itself. But if we don't use those weapons, they certainly won't help us in the war before us. *"No man that warreth entangleth himself with the affairs of this life; that he may please him who hath chosen him to be a soldier. And if a man also strive for masteries, yet is he not crowned, except he strive lawfully. The husbandman that laboreth must be first partaker of the fruits."* (2 Tim. 2:4-6)

Jesus has given the Comforter to those who follow after Him. We, who have the Holy Spirit, have the Spirit of Truth,

Who will guide us unto all truth. *". . . for he shall not speak of himself; but whatsoever he shall hear, that shall he speak: and he will show you things to come. He shall glorify me: for he shall receive of mine, and shall show it unto you!"* (John 16:13-14)

The baptism of the Holy Spirit is a momentous occasion. No matter how good, religious or intellectually spiritualized we may be prior to the coming of the Holy Spirit, we are mere flesh. But when the Holy Spirit comes into us, we are no longer children of this earth of darkness, but we become citizens of the heavenly kingdom. We become children of light. *"For ye were sometimes darkness, but now are ye light in the Lord: walk as children of light: . . . Awake thou that sleepest, and arise from the dead, and Christ shall give thee light."* (Eph. 5:8, 14)

The light of Christ is within us, but if we do not perceive it and look unto it with a single eye, searching to find the glory of God hidden within, will we ever step forth into the fullness of that to which we are called? *"Ye are all children of the light, and the children of the day: we are not of the night, nor of darkness."* (1 Thess. 5:5)

When the Holy Spirit came into us, He became that "outside force" which acted upon the atoms of our physical being, causing the electrons within the atoms to be changed in their orbital path. The vibrations of those atoms were raised and they began orbiting faster and are now producing light, color and sound within our spirits. If you will look within, deep within, past the physical shell, past the sense awareness, past the fount of thought, deep within to the center of your being, you will see the light.

Turning your attention deeply inward, initially, you will perceive perhaps only a small glimmer of light. But if you, day after day, worship Him in spirit and truth, the light will grow until one day it will burst forth bright as the noonday sun. *"This then is the message which we have heard of him, and declare unto you, that God is light, and in him is no darkness at all. But if we walk in the light, as He is in the light, we have fellowship one with another, and the blood of Jesus Christ his Son cleanseth us from all sin."* (1 John 1:5)

Once the light of Christ bursts forth into the mortal mind, we begin to have the mind in us which is in Christ Jesus. I assure you, this light is not a symbolical term used to express spiritualized intellect. This light is a real light. It is brighter than the lamp by which you read. It is brighter than the noonday sun. It is a blue-white light such as you see around the sun at high noon yet it doesn't hurt your eyes or scorch your face when you look upon it. And you cannot encounter even a brief moment of this light, without being lifted up and filled with joy and love, for this light is the glory of God, given *". . . To open their eyes, and to turn them from darkness to light, and from the power of Satan unto God, . . ."* (Acts 26:18)

The one hundred and twenty who awaited the coming of the Comforter in the upper room received the fullness of that Light and Word when *" . . . suddenly there came a sound from heaven as of a rushing mighty wind, and it filled all the house . . . "* (Acts 2:2) They were filled, not only spiritually, but also the inner man and the physical man (the house).

All the divisions of the mind which separate the subconscious of the soul, the conscious of the personality and the super-conscious of the spirit were torn down. The entire mind of each individual was made *one*. Before that moment, they were just like we are now. Their minds were like houses which had a basement, a main floor and an upstairs. Each of the floors had many rooms, closets, nooks and crannies. It is easy to put something away in a house and forget that it is there. It is easy to accumulate a lot of junk in a house with lots of rooms. But, when the Holy Spirit came upon them, the floors separating the basement, the main floor, and the upstairs, all were removed. All the partitions were torn down. Every closet was flung open. Every thought and secret desire was revealed, exposed and washed away under the mighty power of the Holy Spirit. Their minds were made as *one*. One mind instead of three. And, that one mind was made *one* with the mind of Christ.

We have been baptized in the Spirit . . . some of us . . . dunked into the living waters of Light, but we are not filled with the Spirit. *I have not met anyone yet who is filled with the Spirit.* I know some who come under a mighty annointing to do a special work upon occasion but they do not per-petually walk in that annointing. The one man I've met who came closest to being filled with the Spirit was a minister who was a precious and mighty man of God. He had a little church in Pennsylvania. He was filled with the light. You could see it. It made him glow with a translucency not seen in many people. The light shone right through his skin. As he grew older, you could see him diminishing and the light increasing. His physical being just seemed to convert from flesh to light until, toward the end of his life, he seemed to be merely a very thin transparent covering of skin over a body of light. This man didn't speak except to speak for the Lord. He never wasted his power in frivolity. His penetrating eyes saw much about a person but he kept it locked within. He didn't tell anyone what he saw.

He had healing power in his hands but he didn't tell you that either. But you knew he had it because, if he put his hand over you, you felt the power go through your body. If he put his hand over your head, you were lifted up immediately into the spirit and taken to spiritual realms. No one could resist being drawn into the spirit when the power from his hands came into contact with them. He was a precious, dedicated man and anyone who was ever given a prophecy from his spirit could know that he was given the Word of God for his life!

This dear man told me that he received the annointing for a healing ministry after praising God for many hours, daily, for the blessings he had already received. During all those hours of devotion, he would have his hands raised toward heaven, as a symbol of his submission to the will of God. God honored his faithfulness and dedication by giving him the gift of healing in those sacrificed hands.

Jesus said, " . . . *I am the light of the world: he that followeth me shall not walk in darkness, but shall have the light of life!"* (John 8:12) As we follow Him, we will take on His nature.

Following Him means to be like Him, to take on His

nature, to act as He acted, to think as He thought, to speak as He spoke, to love as He loved, to be wholly consecrated unto God the Father as He was wholly consecrated. Is it too soon to take up our cross and follow Him?

"... *If thou knowest the gift of God, and who it is that saith to thee, Give me to drink; thou wouldest have asked of him, and he would have given thee living water.* ... *Whosoever drinketh of this water shall thirst again: But whosoever drinketh of the water that I shall give him shall never thirst; but the water that I shall give him shall be in him a well of water springing up into everlasting life."* (John 4:10, 13-14)

Now the prayer which our Lord Jesus Christ taught us becomes an urgent supplication ... *"Thy will be done in earth, as it is in heaven."* (Matt. 6:10)

Thy "mystery of God" to which Paul alludes so many times in his writings is in the process of being unfolded in this final hour. Those who have been touched by the finger of God are expecting the completion of God's will for man, the will which was been revealed in Eden, in Christ and in heaven. God's will for us is perfection beyond our imagination.

God's Plan is not only for a theocratic government of peace and good will toward all men. His will is that it be on earth, among men, as it is in heaven. He wants to establish His kingdom, the mind of Christ, in us while we yet abide in the flesh. *"Then shall thy light break forth as the morning, and thine health shall spring forth speedily: and thy righteousness shall go before thee; the glory of the Lord shall be thy rearward."* (Isa. 58:8)

Yes, there is a new world coming and it will be beautiful

beyond our wildest expectations and imaginations. *"But as it is written, Eye hath not seen, nor ear heard, neither have entered into the heart of man, the things which God hath prepared for them that love him."* (1 Cor. 2:9)

So it is, all around the world, a person here, another there, feels a deep consecration within to do more in the name of Christ than man has dared dream. I see it in members of my own home congregation, among the evangelicals, the Catholics, the main-line Protestant churches, among those who were orthodox Jews and among those who, just a short time ago, were walking the way of the worldly. *"Now to him that is of power to stablish you according to my gospel, and the preaching of Jesus Christ, according to the revelation of the mystery, which was kept secret since the world began, But now is made manifest, and by the scriptures of the prophets, according to the commandment of the everlasting God, made known to all nations for the obedience of faith: . . . "* (Rom. 16:25-26)

We are called, not only to be a part of this new world, but to help establish it by learning obedience even as Jesus learned obedience. Then will we be able to observe within ourselves that which was seen and recorded by John the Beloved, *"And the city had no need of the sun, neither of the moon, to shine in it: for the glory of God did lighten it, and the Lamb is the light thereof."* (Rev. 21:23)

12

"Wilt Thou Be Made Whole?"

"Now there is at Jerusalem by the sheep market a pool, which is called in the Hebrew tongue Bethesda, having five porches. In these lay a great multitude of impotent folk, of blind, halt, withered, waiting for the moving of the water. For an angel went down at a certain season into the pool, and troubled the water: whosoever then first after the troubling of the water stepped in was made whole of whatsoever disease he had. And a certain man was there, which had an infirmity thirty and eight years. When Jesus saw him lie, and knew that he had been now a long time in that case, he saith unto him, 'Wilt thou be made whole?'" (John 5:2-6)

We, too, have been a long time at the pool, waiting for the angel to trouble the waters so we can step in and be cleansed of all our diseases. The pool at Bethesda reminds me of Moses' well in Midian. Moses engaged in contemplating at the well. He looked into himself to discover who he was so he could better prepare for the call of God upon his life.

At the pool of Bethesda we wait for the angel to trouble the waters.

The angel represents our spirit self. When we have a need which cannot be answered by physical means, the spirit stirs up the waters of the subconscious mind (which is the mind of the soul) and brings to the surface of our awareness the truth which will free us. But we need to step into that pool. We will never be healed if we lie around on one of the five porches — trying to find the answer to our affliction through one of the five senses. We have to be willing to be submerged in the knowledge which springs forth from the soul.

The pool at Bethesda must have been busier than a doctor's office on Monday morning. The place was crowded every day with those who eagerly waited on the edge of the pool. At the first sign of a troubling of the waters they would jump in to get healed. Do you know people like that? They do not wait, for years, hoping to get better, watching others receive their healings while they continue on in their misery. They jump right in at the first sign of trouble and seek out the cause within so they can come into balance with God once again.

There was no one to put this afflicted man into the water. There is no one to help you or me either. Even if we had all kinds of servants, commanded great respect, had great wealth at our disposal or gave orders to large armies, they could not help us get into the troubled waters and discover the source of our infirmity. We each have to come to this point of reality on our own.

Jesus came by and asked, *". . . Wilt thou be made whole?"* Perhaps that seems like a redundant question. After all, the man had been waiting there for a long time. At least that is what he said. But Jesus knew what he was asking because Jesus knew that some people really don't want to be healed. They like the pay-off they get for being ill. They like the attention and the pity and the flowers and get-well cards. They like getting out of work and responsibility. They like having an excuse for lying around in housecoat or robe, smelling of medicine and revelling in self-pity. They like having something to talk about as they recount their symptoms, the lab reports, and their most recent encounter with the spectre of death.

The afflicted man doesn't give Jesus an honest, direct answer to His question. Jesus asked, *" . . . Wilt thou be made whole?"* and the man offers an excuse for being afflicted so long, because he knows in his spirit exactly what Jesus is asking him. So he says, "It isn't really my fault that I have this affliction and have been in bondage for 38 years. I don't have a servant to put me in the water. You see how difficult it is for me. As soon as I get up and start moving toward the water, all the others go in ahead of me. They get the healing and there is nothing left for me."

We all have excuses, don't we? We have come a long way together since the first page of this book. We have considered the ways in which we have made ourselves sick — how we have maintained a state of dis-ease and ill health, just like this man in Bethesda. And we have learned how we have prevented the Lord from making us whole. We, too, have offered excuses as weak justification for our failure to do as we should have done. We have considered the ways in which we can cooperate with the Holy Spirit in making all things new, in order that we can begin to manifest health and well-being in our physical bodies — an outgrowth of the spiritual harmony we have achieved with our Father God. We have learned that, above all else, whenever we fall into ill health, it is our responsibility to examine ourselves carefully to see if we still are "in the faith."

Then Jesus looked deep into his eyes . . . that deep penetrating examination which goes beyond the surface into the uttermost corners of our innermost parts . . . and He put an end to the nonsense, the alibis, the evasions, the delusions and He spoke to the spirit of man, *"Wilt thou be made whole?"*

In that moment, the spirit of the man, at the pool of Bethesda, was called forth to exercise its authority over the personality, to establish balance and harmony throughout the man's entirety, to put away former things, and to become a new creature. Jesus spoke further, *". . . take up thy bed, . . . "* Matt. 9:6.

We have to do something to prove to the personality that faith works. We have to do it without question and without rational understanding. We have to move into untried areas, regardless of how the situation appears. We have to put an end to *wanting to be sick.* We have to take up our beds. We have to be done with them.

"And walk!" To walk is to take a step at a time. From here to there. And from there to beyond. But even a journey around the world begins with a single step. That single step is an application of faith. It is moving out into what we believe to be true until we prove that it *is* true. And as soon as we are willing to go that far, we, just as that man at Bethesda, will be made whole. And no matter what day of the week it is, it will be a Sabbath unto us for we will worship the Father in spirit and in truth!

Jesus then said to the man, *". . . Behold, thou art made whole: sin no more, lest a worse thing come unto thee."* (John 5:14) This man's hidden sin had kept him bound for 38 years. Jesus forgave his sin and told him to sin no more or he would have a worse ailment come unto him. Jesus didn't say he was possessed of devils or foul spirits of infirmity. He didn't say the man had been attacked by Satan. He said, *"Sin no more lest a worse thing come unto thee."*

And as soon as the man went away to give testimony, he was deluged by the Jews — the religious people of the temple who were quick to find fault with what Jesus had done, to cast dispersions on the miracle, to stir up doubt and condemnation, and to offer to the man an explanation of how it should have been done.

We have the "Jews" among us today. Some of them are the conservatives who don't want to change anything from the old ways. They would rather do nothing than to try something new in faith.

There is another type rampant today, too. *"And therefore did the Jews persecute Jesus, and sought to slay him, because he had done these things on the sabbath day."* (John 5:16)

Jesus here represents the highest manifestation of the

Spirit of God known to mankind . . . the Christ! The Christ abides without pause or interruption in a perpetual Sabbath, a time eternal of worshipping God Almighty in the spirit. When the Christ moves, divine healing takes place . . . immediately, and thoroughly, because The Christ sees that perfect Image in which we are made. The Christ can look into our eyes and instantly call forth that divine perfection within us. We are made whole!

We have, today, teachers, preachers, healers and evangelists who are acting out the part of those who persecuted Jesus and sought to slay Him. They don't mean to do that. They do it because they are misinformed. They are dynamic, charismatic, hypnotic, inspiring, motivating and convincing. They recite Scriptures which they do not understand. They do not wait to be taught of the Holy Spirit. So they teach false doctrine which seeks to slay the divine perfection of Christ! They follow the written Word instead of the *Spirit* of the written Word.

Appearing like clones, their message is a mimeographed, tape-recorded copy of one teaching which sounds so right you wonder why no one ever thought of it sooner. But, this teaching can be extremely dangerous. It is important to follow the *Spirit* of the written Word, not just the "written" Word alone. We need to let the Holy Spirit *illumine* the Word to our hearts. This takes the discipline of reading the Word and meditating upon it — absorbing it into our very beings.

Although, we know that God can make anything out of anybody, the people about which we speak are, in my opinion, not likely to make the Word applicable to their daily lives. They do not take the time to PROVE THE WORD! They teach *concepts* instead of wisdom. They teach "parts" of the Word instead of the *whole* Word.

A few months ago, I heard one of these well-known teachers say that if you had faith, you wouldn't go to a doctor. If you had faith, you wouldn't take that insulin. If you had faith, you would throw away that high blood pressure medicine. *"And therefore did the Jews persecute Jesus, . . . "* (John 5:16)

IF THE LORD HAS HEALED YOU OF YOUR AIL-MENT, *HE* WILL TELL YOU WHEN YOU NO LONGER NEED THAT PRESCRIPTION! Don't *dare* throw away your medicine! People have died that way. You can't be healed on someone else's faith! You have to be the one who has gone down into the pool of healing. And you can sit *by* the pool for 38 years but that won't heal you either. It has to be a personal experience of your own! And when it is, you will be the first one to know about it!

For over ten years I had a thyroid imbalance, for which I had to take five grains of thyroxin daily. The imbalance was caused by a misuse of the power given me to use. I spent too much of the power trying to balance my life between what other people expected of me and what I knew God wanted me to do. I was not developed fully in my personal-ity, so I was constantly permitting others to put me in bondage. I had seen the angel come down and trouble the water and I had gone into the water to be made whole but hadn't been ready for it at all levels of consciousness. I wasn't really ready to trust the Lord completely by following Him without reservation, because I was defying the people who were trying to keep me in captivity.

Then Jesus spoke to me with a loving but piercing look and asked, *"Wilt thou be made whole?"* "Yes," I said. "I'm ready, but what will these people in my life who want to control me say?" And Jesus said, *"You follow me and I'll take care of them."* (Paraphrased) I was healed. I knew it. I believed with all my heart that I was healed. But I continued to take the medicine until I felt God speaking to my heart that I no longer needed it.

I remember the exact hour when I knew when it was no longer necessary. I left work, drove twenty miles to the doctor, told him I believed I had been healed and no longer needed the medication. He ordered tests at the hospital and the results showed that I was healed. My thyroid was in perfect balance and I could discontinue the medicine.

In my opinion, it is more likely that God will speak directly to you concerning your own body. Why would God tell a perfect stranger, who has come to town to conduct revival meetings, something about your health, something He has neglected to tell you? Does that make sense? Wouldn't it be more practical for the Lord to reveal it to you since it does concern your own health? Just because an evangelist has had a "word of knowledge" for you doesn't mean, by any stretch of the imagination, that he knows what is wrong with your innermost parts and how to get them fixed. Be sensible. God gave you a mind for a reason!

I have travelled to distant cities and observed some of

these evangelists who have risen out of obscurity to become nationally known as "great healers." Unfortunately, some of them had all the earmarks of sideshow barkers. They created an atmosphere of emotional frenzy. Anything was possible in the midst of that reservoir of human magnetism. But what happened when the people left the meeting? Many of them sank right back to where they had been before they came. *". . . , and sought to slay him, because he had done these things on the sabbath day."* (John 5:16)

Let me explain — we humans have the potential to build tremendous power within ourselves. Those who are adept at this power can build up a tremendous store of it which can be used to achieve what they wish. It is that power which makes great actors, politicians, lecturers, musicians, hypnotists, performers, athletes, doctors, evangelists and healers. It is the power of magnetism. It is not the power from on high. *"But Jesus answered them, My Father worketh hitherto, and I work."* (John 5:17)

Magnetism can be transferred from one person to another. Those who know about it can draw it from the earth, the air, the sun, the crowd.

Those who know how to utilize it, can feel when it is coming into them and when it is going out. They can direct it where they want it to make it do what they want. Remember what I said earlier about the power from on high? *The difference is where this power comes from.*

Magnetic power is stimulated and increased by the EMOTIONS. It comes into the body anywhere from the waist down, generally stirring first in the abdominal region and sending out waves of energy which we often call shivers, goose flesh, dodads, or joy bumps down toward our feet and back up again. Sometimes we can feel our bodies drawing in this magnetic power from the crowds or from our surroundings.

Many of those who claim to be healers fall into the category of magnetic healing. They are able to transfer, to another person, an oversupply of energy which they have produced, gathered and stored within their own bodies. It can be compared to giving a jump to a car whose battery is run down. But even as the car with the weakened battery can run for a time on the shot of power it received from a healthy battery, a weakened body can do the same thing. The problem is that, unless measures are taken in the ailing body to bring it to health, that little "battery jump" isn't going to suffice for a very long time. That is why some people think they receive a healing when they come under the influence of such a healer. Temporarily, they *are* better, but THEY ARE NOT HEALED!

When that shot of power they received from the magnetic healer runs down, they return to the state of disease or ill health which they had prior to the meeting. *How can you tell a magnetic healer from a spiritual healer? . . . by his fruits.*

I recently attended the meeting of a famous healer whom I would relegate to the category of magnetic power. He stirred the crowd with every kind of emotional ploy possible. After he had the multitude clinging to the edge of frenzy the healing service began. There were those who gave up crutches and back braces, others who walked when they could scarcely crawl prior to the meeting, those who ran when before they could barely walk. But I was not convinced that any of those people were permanently healed.

"Therefore the Jews sought the more to kill him, because he not only had broken the sabbath, but said also that God was his Father, making himself equal with God." (John 5:18)

We are told to discern the spirits, are we not? In 1965 I began observing and collecting data on healers and healings. I have received a countless number of healings for myself, my family, and friends.

Many of the "magnetic healers" do not use the Word of God in their meetings. They use gimmicks which stimulate a strong emotional response in the audience. They stimulate fear . . . the world is coming to an end, the tribulation is about to take place, the coming of the Lord is at hand. They use sentiment, guilt, elation, jubilation, even overt adoration and praise — anything that stimulates a strong emotional response in the group.

When a large group of people all begin to experience the same emotion, it produces a supply of energy sufficient for any purpose. If we had the equipment to measure energy, we would be amazed at the intensity. But, this is only human magnetism.

There is a price on the work of the magnetic healer. He makes no apologies about it. This is one time when he doesn't hold back quoting Scripture. *". . . for the workman is worthy of his meat."* (Matt. 10:10) This man or woman can quickly put an audience into bondage with guilt if the offering is not what they expected. They pull lots of gimmicks in this area, too, in order to get the money. Such as,

"The Lord has just spoken to me that there are ten persons in this audience who are each going to give a thousand dollars. God is not a liar. Who are those ten persons? Don't turn a deaf ear to the Lord. Hold up that check! Let's give a wave offering to the Lord!"

Such shenanigans make the Word and work of God look like charlatanry. It makes those who believe look like fools. *"Then answered Jesus and said unto them, Verily, verily, I say unto you, The Son can do nothing of himself, but what he seeth the Father do: for what things soever he doeth, these also doeth the Son likewise."* (John 5:19)

Obviously, these men are not getting their direction from the Lord. I wish we didn't have them out front making so much commotion, but they abounded in the time of the apostles, and there are even more of them today. We as believers, should spot them. We should be very discerning about where we give gifts and offerings to the Lord. Is it furthering the work of our Lord by spreading the gospel, or is it furthering the aims of some self-proclaimed evangelists who see a good opportunity to fleece the flock?

I have been in services where I was convinced that the power which was used to bring about the miracles was of Divine origin. Cases were documented and proven through medical means. These are the signs of which Jesus spoke.

There are many new ministries in the area of healing who just are not experienced enough to understand the modus operandi involved in spiritual healing. They make mistakes as an apprentice makes mistakes. But they are open to learn and to be led. We need prayer warriors to intercede on behalf of these new ministries. They will be perfected as long as they pray to stay in the center of God's perfect will.

Spiritual healing is as different from magnetic healing as a saint is different from a fortune teller. The people who are used in this area are different also. You can feel the difference in them as soon as you come into their presence. Power fairly emanates from them. These are people who are "spiritual giants," and they didn't become "spiritual giants" overnight. They have known who they are in Christ. They have lived dedicated lives of service and submission to God. They have the Word in them, and they abide in the Word. They have made many sacrifices in order to become vessels of honor unto the Lord. Kathryn Kuhlman was such a person. When she walked into an auditorium you knew she was there, even if you didn't see her, because she emanated such tremendous power and light. If she reached out to shake hands with you, you fell under the power. Yet she claimed nothing for herself or of herself. She repeatedly and emphatically declared that she was not a healer. And she conducted her services in such a manner that a person could not confuse the issue. Still, there were those who went away saying they were healed by Kathryn Kuhlman.

She didn't call people down to the front so she could lay hands on them. She knew that it was the Holy Spirit who did the work and He worked in the auditorium among the people. He moved freely up and down the rows, touching those who were ready to let go of their infirmity, and Miss Kuhlman ministered through the *word of knowledge.* She did everything she could to minimize her part in the service, so that all praise, honor and glory went where it belonged . . . to God. So many would-be healers unwittingly bring the attention to themselves rather than God. Consequently, they force the withdrawal of the Holy Spirit. *"But I have a greater witness than that of John: for the works which the Father hath given me to finish, the same works that I do, bear witness of me, that the Father hath sent me."* (John 5:36)

Spiritual power is a higher energy than magnetic power. It is produced, not by emotionalism, but by devotion and love. It works through the soul of the individual rather than the personality or physical vehicle. It is generated in the area of the heart, and when it is released moves upward to the head.

The Scriptures tell us that gifts of healing are available to believers through the Holy Spirit. Many people want to serve God and have power in their lives. But they must search the Scriptures and learn the difference between a true gift and that which is false. I have known people who are necromancers, in every degree of the word, who have laid on hands, for healing, and unknowledgeable people believe they are "spiritual." They are not spiritual. They are *spiritistic* — which is to say they are dealing in the area of the black arts and are using magnetism rather than the power of God. Many are drawn into the occult, in such a manner, and never realize what has happened to them . . . until it is too late.

Spiritual power cannot be produced or maintained by anyone who does not possess the fruits of the spirit. We should avoid anyone who introduces himself as a "healer," but is obviously lacking the fruits. Don't give him your gifts or offerings. Don't give him your nodding encouragement. Don't do anything to further his work, because he is not doing this work for God. He is doing it for self. *"But I know you that ye have not the love of God in you."* (John 5:42)

The prime spiritual fruit necessary to produce spiritual power is, of course, love . . . love of the higher self, love for God and love for fellowman. It must be a sincere love developed in the soul which cares and burdens for the plights of others; a love which senses the need of others to such a degree that when a brother suffers, he suffers. This kind of love is not developed from the outside. It is developed from the level of soul. Either it is within that soul to have compassion and mercy or it is not. And one who has that degree of humanity does what is necessary in order to serve his brothers. It is not so much a decision he makes as it is a calling to which he responds. Then, whatever he must lay down of personal desire, in order to fulfill this calling, counts not as loss, because personal desire is not that important to him. He knows, within his heart, that in order to really live, he must serve mankind. And he does not do it for recognition or remuneration. Instead, he does it because it is the only way he knows to live. Mother Theresa, *Nobel Peace Prize* winner, is that kind of person. Dr. Albert Schweitzer was another, and Dr. Tom Dooley, and Mark Buntain. Praise God! There are so many *great oaks of strength* planted on earth who encourage us when we have just about lost all human hope.

Spiritual power is developed quietly and automatically as the natural outgrowth of great spiritual devotion, dedication and submission. It grows in a person who is not looking to develop it because he doesn't have time to have his eyes upon himself. He is busy taking care of the needs of those about him.

Recently, I heard some young Christians speaking about "coveting the gifts." These youth were "scriptural" but naive. There is a price to pay for spiritual gifts, and those who have these gifts have paid a great price. Why would a newcomer receive these gifts when he hasn't even made initial sacrifices of physical lusts and ego attachments?

Divine power comes from on high. It needs only the faith of the believer who is calling upon it for it to manifest. It can work through the most common persons when God chooses to use them. It can work against any odds at any time, in any place. And when this power comes, all darkness, negativity, disease or sickness of any kind must bow before its majesty.

When the power of the Holy Spirit comes into the human body, it comes down through the top of the head and the presence of it automatically lifts the consciousness of the individual up into the spiritual realm. This power sometimes is accompanied by a brilliant light and by a force which feels like electricity.

When God's healing power comes into a person, whether directly from the Lord or through another person who is serving as a channel, the healing is complete. The reason for that is because the spirit of the individual is healed first. Once all trace of iniquity is cleansed from the spirit, the body must duplicate its pattern. That is why Jesus said, *" . . . Behold, thou art made whole: sin no more, lest a worse thing come unto thee."* (John 5:14) Seeing the spiritual cause of the affliction, Jesus could look into the hidden recesses of the person and call out that secret or forgotten sin which started the affliction in the body. He could speak, in power, to the spirit and soul of that person saying, "You are forgiven," and the afflicted person could, in that moment, be free of all memory of that transgression.

Not knowing the cause of a person's affliction is the main reason the healer does not get positive results from his prayer of faith. He didn't know what to ask for when he prayed so he didn't get positive results. An example is that of a retarded adult who was brought forth at a service for healing. The prayer was for the demons to come out of him!

Over the past ten years, I have worked with a number of retarded adults, and I have never yet met one that even vaguely resembled a demoniac or was influenced by foul spirits. The retarded adults I have known have been beautiful, innocent souls who are more like angels than demons. I say this with all sincerity. I have come to love retarded persons. They lack guile and have sweetness of spirit, openness, and a lack of deceit. They are retarded because of brain damage or defects in the brain during gestation. Some retardation may occur because of lack of proper care during infancy. But I do not believe that retardation is the result of demonic possession or the influence of "foul spirits."

What will happen to the afflicted if we do not pray with spiritual understanding, and according to God's will? Nothing. and their faith may be injured because others might say either the church is on the wrong track or healing is not for today.

Do not pray for healing for one who has not asked for it. It is good to have compassion on the suffering and limitations of another person. But that does not mean that we shall get healing results for them.

One evening as my husband and I were waiting at a railroad crossing, a young man approached who was severely handicapped with a crippling disease such as multiple sclerosis. His twisted legs teetered at the edge of the track and I sat poised to jump out of the car to grab him by his shirt tail should he begin to fall toward the clanking wheels of the train. I was so moved with compassion for this young man that I began to grieve in the spirit, crying out, "Oh God! I pray that I could have the power such as Jesus had to just point my finger at that boy and have him made whole and straight!"

My husband tenderly held me for a moment and spoke wisely to my grief, "Jesus had that kind of power but he did not heal every one who was afflicted, Joyce. He healed only those who were going to be helped by the healing. The others had to remain as they were!"

I suddenly realized how true that was. Jesus could have gone through the cities and villages healing everyone. Surely he had the compassion to do so. He could have completely eradicated sickness from the face of the earth. But he healed only those who asked for the healing and those who were spiritually prepared to let go of their affliction.

Some ministries have an open and blanket acceptance that every person who comes forth for healing of any kind of affliction has been taken over by some kind of demon or foul spirit. I doubt that if they even met someone with a demon or foul spirit they would try to call it out. More likely, they would run in the opposite direction. Casting out demons requires spiritual guidance.

The more I observe the floundering of new ministries in the area of healing the more I am convinced that if we are going to work in this area of signs and wonders we should first ask for the Lord to give us the gift of discerning of spirits. I don't mean "spiritual discernment." That is something else.

The discerning of spirits is the ability to see not only into the spiritual realm where demons and devils abound but also to discern the spirit of the individual asking for healing. Without that we cannot have wisdom concerning that person. With the indwelling of the Holy Spirit we will know how to make intercession on behalf of that person. For instance, if a person comes forth for healing of arthritis a discernment of that person's spirit may reveal that the hardness and swelling of the bones and joints is due to a wrong mental or emotional attitude. They may have a heart full of bitterness and resentment toward another person whom they might feel has wronged them. They are tolerating that person's actions while resenting it inside. The resentment causes the Ph level of the system to become so unbalanced that the joints begin to ache and swell. They are not aware that the hidden resentment is a stumbling block to their relationship with the Lord. They are aware only of the pain. Would it be according to the purpose of God for that person to receive healing of the physical condition when the heart is in a state of disharmony? Of course not! So the prayer for healing is not answered. The congregation sees that and their faith is injured.

Often, those who are adept at making excuses will quickly come back with the statement, "Oh but she was healed of that arthritis! God healed her but she didn't receive." This is not true. When the resentment is gone, when the personal life is brought under the blood of Jesus Christ, when all unforgiveness is released, the healing will be complete.

There is a famous healer who lays hands on people and commands, "Oh foul spirit of nicotine, come out" – regardless of the reason the person came forth for healing. Apparently, he can see that they have an addiction to tobacco. But just because he commands that spirit to leave doesn't mean that it will. If the possessor of that spirit doesn't want it to leave his body temple why would the demon leave?

You can't make a person make sacrifices of carnal things just because you think they should.

Many times those who are called to serve through the gifts of the Spirit at first are open to the leading of the Lord. Later, they forsake His teaching and follow the ways of others. Lacking spiritual understanding, they do what they see others do. Soon, the annointing is lifted, and they are left to flounder on their own, not because of the unfaithfulness of the Lord, but because they did not wait upon Him. They got impatient and began adding their own ideas to the wisdom of God.

Those who are called into a healing ministry will be *annointed* by the Lord. They will be taught, led, tested and tried as they are prepared to be a useful instrument of the Lord. They will need to go through fire to be made strong enough to take the criticism and abuse which is sure to follow. They will be proved by the Lord to be sincere and strong enough to withstand temptation and tribulation. Do you think it is just as easy as taking a Scripture out of context, and saying, "I am a believer so I will lay hands on the sick and they will recover." Ridiculous! With the high cost of medical treatment today, don't you think we would all be laying hands on people if it were that easy?

It takes power to heal, and the vessel has to be appropriate for the power. It isn't easy to be any kind of vessel for the Lord. It wasn't intended to be easy. Only the most fervent and sincere will survive. The Lord knows that those who remain faithful, regardless of all shipwrecks, beatings, stonings, and imprisonments, are those who love Him enough to serve Him, whatever the cost.

That is why some, who begin this journey with sincerity, are deceived before they finish the journey. They become so bogged down with worldly cares about money, debts, responsibilities, time schedules, and personal illness, that they forget their first love. Then, they begin to seek their own profit. When I see this, the spirit in me becomes so grieved that I can do nothing but pray in the Spirit in intercession for them.

As we go through our apprenticeship . . . even as Moses did with the rod of power . . . we learn how the Lord works, how He speaks, how it feels when He is annointing us, when He is leading us . . . and sometimes through trial and error . . . we learn to become totally surrendered in His hands. We know, beyond the shadow of a doubt, that it is He who does the works and not us. Until we have that inner enlightenment we are working out of self and can do no good thing. Only the Spirit of the Lord in us can do it.

Sometimes, however, the Lord doesn't give us what we ask. Regardless of what some would tell you, it is not always God's plan to answer your prayer in the affirmative, either when you pray for another or when you are asking healing for yourself. By that I do not mean that it is ever God's will for a person to suffer from some debilitating illness. God's will for all of us, at all times, is perfect peace and we cannot have that peace when we are suffering.

God can heal us but He doesn't always choose to do so when we ask. It may be, as stated in an earlier chapter, that there are lessons which must first be gleaned from the circumstances in which we find ourselves. Or perhaps, it is in that situation where we will learn that which will bring glory to God.

From where we sit, with our noses pressed against the tapestry of our lives, we cannot see the design which God is creating. We see only that which is within the range of our natural vision. When we are so close to it the colors and designs are blurred and indefinable. But from a distance, sometimes in retrospect, we see how His glory shines through our darkest hours.

The automobile accident I experienced taught me so many things and made me available for God to use. While I was still in *intensive care,* in the midst of my pain, I was able to lead a suicide victim to Christ before she died, and to comfort a night-duty nurse who had only weeks before lost a teen-age son to leukemia.

I believe that a child of God should never lose sight of who he is — regardless of his circumstances. If you, as a born-again believer, should be overcome with an illness, it is self-centered to start wailing, "Why me, Lord?" and then begin to worry about what someone else is going to say. If you have prayed to be used of God no matter what the cost, why can't you take that illness as just another opportunity to serve Him? Have you any idea how many times it can work out in that manner if you will only turn your eyes toward Him and away from self?

I have never had a situation in my entire life which didn't, in the final analysis, glorify God. It is a waste of precious God given energy to begin worrying about what someone is going to think if I fall prey to sickness or weakness. Sure, they talk and mock and criticise. So what? Haven't we been told that in this world we are always going to have tribulation? Regardless of what befalls me, I am going to seek for the *Holy Grail* in the midst of that experience and God will get the credit and the glory for every wonderful thing I learn while I am there. That way, my eyes, from the outset, will be open to discover the ways in which I can serve God right where I am. That is the manner in which the Lord has taught me. It hasn't been by tablets of stone handed down from heaven. It has been in the midst of my error.

A born-again believer may be bringing about his affliction through any one of the means which we covered throughout this book. He should seek the wisdom of God concerning his affliction so that he may be done with this lesson once and for all time.

But, even as he is humbling himself before the Lord and confessing his error, he can turn his mind around and see the double-fold purpose of the illness as God's opportunity to fulfill His purpose of:

1. *Purification* 2. *Sanctification* 3. *Wisdom* 4. *Compassion* 5. *Justification*

Jesus began his miraculous ministry during the wedding at Cana. After that, Jesus went to a feast of the Jews in Jerusalem.

Remember, Cana represents the spiritual power latent in the spoken Word. The wedding was representative of the spirit and personality working together for the glory of God. Jerusalem is the Holy City, representing a state of consciousness, in which we may continually abide if we keep our eyes singularly affixed on the risen Christ. The Jew represents the religious ideas of spiritualized intellect — there was a celebration, a feast of the spiritualized consciousness.

When we experience the power of God, either working in us to heal us, or working through us to heal another, there is celebration. Our minds are filled with the knowledge of how the Word of God can be brought into manifestation. In those moments, when His presence is so real to us, we receive an instant panoramic view of the purpose and plan of God. Then we know, without a shadow of doubt, *". . . ALL things are possible for those who love God"* (Mark 10:27 Paraphrased), and we can say with Paul, *"For our light affliction, which is but for a moment, worketh for us a far more exceeding and eternal weight in glory; . . . "* (2 Cor. 4:17)

Go and tell the good news. Shout it from the housetops! *"And be ready always to give an answer to every man that asketh you a reason of the hope that is in you with meekness and fear: . . . "* (1 Pet. 3:15)

The more you look for signs of God's handiwork in your life, the more you will find them and the greater your faith will be. The more your faith grows, the more you will love the Lord; the more you love Him, the more refined your soul will become. And through this love, will begin the refining process which will prepare you to receive. Not only will you be made whole, you will be used to help others, who stand today where you stood yesterday.

We come before Jesus now; limping, halt, blind, maimed — inwardly and outwardly. Our faces are tear-stained from the grief we have silently borne. We, too, have left crimson stains in the sands of time from our scourgings, even though no one has benefitted from our shed blood. Many of us have dragged our rough-hewn crosses along the *Way of Sorrows.* But always there was that hope within that somehow, some-day, we would meet the Master by the wayside, and He would reach out His hand of mercy to heal us. Now, as we push our way through the multitude and come closer to Him, as we heave against the crush of the crowd to come into His presence . . . now, when His eyes light upon us and we cry out, "Jesus! Master! Heal me!" He asks in arresting honesty, *"Wilt thou be made whole?"*

He *always* asks that question, whether we encounter Him in the privacy of our prayer closets, or in the hospital, or in the midst of the multitude. . . . *"Wilt thou be made whole?"* He asks when we go to Him for comfort. It is our decision — *wholeness or fragmentation. Being wholly possessed of God means we share His kingdom of health, happiness, wisdom, prosperity, and spirituality.* To be fragmented is to be divided between God and Satan, good and evil, heaven and hell, the Spirit and the world — where we drag along our sickness, discord, and financial problems.

"Wilt thou be made whole?" Will you give up selfishness, pride, egotism and resentment? Will you release from your prison of memory that one who has wronged you? Will you forgive and forget all your yesterdays and receive His gift of New Life?

He stretches forth His healing hand and again asks, *"Wilt thou be made whole? . . ."*

BIBLIOGRAPHY

Arehart-Treichel, Joan, *Bio-Types,* Times Books, New York, N.Y. 1980

Alexander, Franz, *Psychosomatic Medicine: Its Principles And Applications,* W.W. Norton, New York, N.Y. 1950

Andrews, Lewis M. and Karlins, Marvin, *Biofeedback: Turning On The Power Of Your Mind,* Warner Books, Inc., New York, N.Y. 1973

Bible, King James Version, Thomas Nelson, Inc., Nashville, Tenn. 1978

Bible, Revised Standard Version, Collins-World, Cleveland, 1946-1952

Bucke, Richard M. M.D., *Cosmic Consciousness,* E.P. Dutton & Co., New York, N.Y. 1969

Dunbar, Helen Flanders, *Emotions And Bodily Changes,* Columbia University Press, New York, N.Y. 1954

Dunbar, Helen Flanders, *Psychosomatic Diagnosis,* Paul Hoeber, New York, N.Y. 1943

Dunbar, Helen Flanders, *Mind And Body: Psychosomatic Medicine,* Random House, New York, N.Y. 1966

Epp, Theodore H., *The Other Comforter,* Back to the Bible, Lincoln, Neb. 1966

Gallagher, Richard, *Diseases That Plague Modern Man,* Oceana Publications, Dobbs Ferry, N.Y. 1969

Gibran, Kahlil, *The Prophet,* Alfred A. Knopf, New York, N.Y. 1972

Jacobson, Edith, *Depression,* International University Press, Inc., New York, N.Y. 1971

Jacobi, Jolande, *The Psychology Of C. G. Jung,* Yale University Press, New Haven, 1962

James, William, *The Varieties Of Religious Experience,* New York, Mentor Books, 1958

Jones, E. Stanley, *The Way To Power And Poise,* Abingdon-Cokesbury Press, New York, N.Y., Nashville, Tenn. 1949

Jung, C. G., *Modern Man In Search Of A Soul,* Translated by W.S. Dell and C.F. Baynes, New York, N.Y. and London, England

Jung, C. G., *Psychology And Religion,* Yale University Press, New Haven, 1938

Jung, C. G., *The Development Of Personality,* Collected Works of C. G. Jung, Pantheon Books, Inc., New York, N.Y. 1954

Kugler, Hans J., *Slowing Down The Aging Process,* Pyramid Books, New York, N.Y. 1973

Lawrence, Brother, *The Practice Of The Presence Of God,* Peter Pauper Press, Mount Vernon, N.Y. 1963

Lewis, Howard R. and Martha E., *Psychosomatics,* Viking Press, New York, N.Y. 1972

Menninger, Karl, *The Vital Balance,* Viking Press, New York, N.Y. 1963

Neal, Emily Gardiner, *God Can Heal You Now,* Prentice-Hall, Inc., Englewood Cliffs, N.J. 1958

O'Brien, Elmer, *Varieties Of Mystic Experience,* Mentor-Omega Books, New York, N.Y. 1964

Progoff, Ira, *The Cloud Of Unknowing,* Dell Publishing Co., Inc., New York, N.Y. 1957

Pusey, Edward B., *The Confessions Of Saint Augustine,* Collier Books, New York, N.Y. 1961

Rapaport, Howard & Linde, Shirley M., *"The Complete Allergy Guide,"* Simon and Schuster, New York, N.Y. 1970

Schep, John A., *Baptism In The Spirit,* Logos International, Plainfield, N.J. 1972

Shaw, Linda, *Break Away From Fear,* Prevention Magazine, May 1980, Rodale Press, Emmaus, Pa.

Watson, George, *Nutrition And Your Mind,* Harper and Row, New York; Fitzhenry & Whiteside Limited, Toronto 1972

Whitman Walt, *Leaves Of Grass,* Signet Classics, New York, N.Y. 1955

Wuest, Kenneth S., *Studies In The Vocabulary Of The Greek New Testament,* Wm. B. Eerdmans Publishing Co., Grand Rapids, Mich. 1945

SCRIPTURE REFERENCES

CHAPTER 1

Rom. 13:11-12	James 5:14
Matt. 21:21	Matt. 21:22
Mark 9:23	Mark 11:24
Matt. 13:31	Acts 3:4
Rom. 8:28	2 Cor. 4:17
2 Tim. 4:3	2 Tim. 2:3
2 Tim. 4:5	Heb. 12:5
James 5:10	1 Pet. 4:12
1 Pet 4:19	1 Pet. 5:6
James 4:15	James 4:10
Rom. 8:21-23	Rev. 21:4
Psa. 199:75	Neh. 9:33
Ex. 15	Dan. 9:14
Mic. 7:9	Luke 23:40
Acts 13	1 Cor. 11
James 5:14	Rom. 5:12
James 1:14	Psa. 38:3
Rom. 7:5	Psa. 119:71
2 Pet. 2:13a	1 Pet. 2:24
1 Pet. 4:1	1 Pet. 2:24b
Matt. 7:12	Luke 6:31
Gal. 5:14	Psa. 32:8
2 Pet. 1:19b	John 14:12
1 Pet. 4:16-19	John 1:14
Acts 1:8	John 16:13
1 Thess. 1:5	1 Cor. 4:20
Matt. 6:33	Luke 11:20
Matt. 12:25	John 6:40
1 Thess. 4:3-4	Acts 2:1

CHAPTER 2

Ex. 15:26
Phil. 2:15
John 10:10
John 3:30
Isa. 1:16-20

Prov. 3:11
Rom. 8:28
2 Cor. 10:4-6
Isa. 1:5-6
2 Tim. 4:3

CHAPTER 3

Psa. 107:17
2 Thess. 2:15
Phil. 4:7a
Heb. 12:6
Deut. 28:14-15
Deut. 28:20
2 Cor. 4:17
Matt. 5:48
Gal. 6:7-8
Gal. 5:18
Matt. 5:39
Prov. 3:7-8

Psa. 121:1b
1 Cor. 15:58
1 Kings 9:15
Matt. 21:22
Heb. 5:8-9
Ezra 9:13
Matt. 5:18
Rom. 3:31
1 John 5:18
Psa. 1:1-13
Matt. 5:25-26
Rom. 12:1

CHAPTER 4

Eph. 5:15-17
Phil. 2:12-13
Acts 20:28a
Eph. 3:16
1 Tim. 4:7b-10
Eph. 4:22-24
Luke 17:20b-21
2 Cor. 7:10
Acts 26:18
Rom. 12:2
2 Tim. 2:21
James 4:8

James 3:3
Psa. 119:9
Eph. 5:14
Rom. 8:5-8
John 4:23
Matt. 5:3
Ezek. 36:26-28; 11:21
Matt. 7:26
Luke 11:34
2 Chron. 34
1 John 3:2-3
Prov. 23:7

CHAPTER 5

1 Cor. 13:11
Col. 1:12-13
Luke 10:17-18
1 Pet. 3:4
1 Thess. 5:23

Matt. 28:18
Matt. 12:34
Luke 4:1-13
1 John 5:18

CHAPTER 6

Isa. 10:1
Matt. 12:34-35
Job 22:28a
Ex. 3:13

Matt. 12:37
Eph. 4:22, 25, 29
Ecc. 11:1
Ex. 3:14

CHAPTER 9

1 Cor. 15:51
Phil. 3:12-15
Deut. 4:38
2 Cor. 3:17
John 4:23
Nu. 21:8
Nu. 14:9
Ex. 17:14

1 Cor. 15:53-54
Deut. 4:33
Deut. 5:32-33
2 Cor. 4:6-7
2 Cor. 3:18
John 3:14
Nu. 33:53
Matt. 26:41

CHAPTER 10

Isa. 35:8-10
2 Chron. 1:3
Ecc. 1:2
Mark 12:30-31
1 Cor. 15:9
Rom. 13:11

Rom. 13:1-2
Rev. 2:7
John 4:24
Acts 17:28
1 Cor. 13:10

CHAPTER 11

1 Cor. 2:11-16
Matt. 28:18
John 14:13
John 1:6-9
1 Chron. 28:13
Psa. 33:6
Phil. 2:5
Rom. 13:14
1 John 3:3
John 16:13-14
1 Thess. 5:5
Acts 26:18

John 5:30
John 15:7
John 15:4
Gen. 1:3
Job 33:4
Acts 17:25-28
1 Kings 9:15
1 John 3:2
2 Tim. 2:4-6
Eph. 5:8, 14
1 John 1:5
Acts 2:2

CHAPTER 12

John 5:2-6
John 5:14
John 5:17
Matt. 10:10
John 5:36
John 5:14
2 Cor. 4:17

Matt. 9:6
John 5:16
John 5:18
John 5:19
John 5:42
Mark 10:27
1 Pet. 3:15